The Secret Art
of Pressure Point Fighting

The Secret Art of Pressure Point Fighting

Techniques to Disable Anyone in Seconds Using Minimal Force

Vince Morris

Photographs by Bill Bly

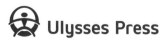 Ulysses Press

Published in the United States by
ULYSSES PRESS
P.O. Box 3440
Berkeley, CA 94703
www.ulyssespress.com

ISBN13: 978-1-56975-623-2
Library of Congress Control Number 2007933419

Printed in Canada by Webcom

10 9 8 7 6 5 4

Acquisitions	Nick Denton-Brown
Editorial/Production	Lily Chou, Claire Chun, Judith Metzener, Steven Zah Schwartz
Index	Sayre Van Young
Design	what!design @ whatweb.com
Cover photograph	© Andy Mogg
Models	Kari Adler, Eva Bayerlein, Matt Knorr, Dan Miller, Debbie Montgomery, Steve Montgomery, Vince Morris, Doug Wachs

Distributed by Publishers Group West

Please Note
This book has been written and published strictly for informational purposes, and in no way should be used as a substitute for actual instruction with qualified professionals. The author and publisher are providing you with information in this work so that you can have the knowledge and can choose, at your own risk, to act on that knowledge. The author and publisher also urge all readers to be aware of their health status and to consult health care professionals before beginning any health or exercise program.

With love and thanks to Eva.

Table of Contents

Foreword

Whatever the lineage of the martial art you practice and study, there is a high probability that the use of pressure points was integrated into the system from the onset. There is ample written and photographic evidence that the Chinese and Okinawan masters, predating the "modern era" of karate I refer to as post-1920s, understood how to leverage weaknesses or features in the human body to their advantage during a fight.

However, as martial arts swept their way from the confines of secret trainings with select membership to a broad general population across the world, attention to the use of these vital points and their roles within the systems was generally diluted or lost. The reasons for this are numerous, but certainly include attempts to make it a sport, World War II, the age and experience of some of the instructors responsible for spreading martial arts, and business aspirations.

My own personal training, now spanning some 30 years, is evidence. I have the utmost respect and admiration for the instructors of the Japan Karate Association who I had the fortunate opportunity to meet up with when attending Drexel University in Philadelphia, PA. They started me on the "way of karate," and they are responsible for much of what is important in my life—family, health and continual character development. Yet in the first 20 years of my training, we never spoke of vital points, never had a class that explained them, nor understood their now-obvious role in the martial arts.

It was this void in part that inspired me to seek more from my training. This activity resulted in the opportunity to cross paths with the author of this book, Vince Morris. I do not exaggerate when I say that the first training sessions with Vince in my dojo changed the way the students in attendance (more than 100 people) viewed martial arts forever. There were many factors responsible, but one at the top of the heap was the incorporation of vital points into the training that none in attendance had experienced before.

I didn't know it at the time, but Vince was in the forefront of a resurrection of information content concerning pressure points. His work began as early as 1978, and has been in refinement ever since.

It is important to note the refinement process. What you will read and learn in this book will not be theories or techniques based on "chi force" or the correct order or time of day to strike a vital point. You will learn what really works when things get nasty. The refinement process has been in the works for many years now and is rooted in countless hours of study, training and practice.

I have been involved with the process for the past ten years, and it has taken Vince and me around the globe. Both martial artists and law enforcement personnel have been exposed to techniques utilizing pressure points; the latter group especially has no time for ineffective technique since their lives may depend on them.

So read on, learn the value of pressure points, and understand that unto themselves they are limited, but coupled with quality technique and the wisdom in this book, they are vital!

Steve Montgomery
7th Dan, Chief Instructor
Kissaki-Kai Karate-do
Cherry Hill, NJ
March 2008

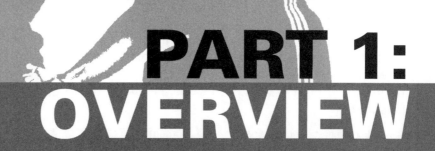

PART 1:
OVERVIEW

Introduction

It would be dishonest of me to present this book as if the vital points, and how they can facilitate the defeat of an attacker in combat situations, were simple to understand, learn and apply. In my seminars, I remind participants that knowledge of kyusho jutsu ("the art of vital points") is as useful in combat as applying poison to the tip of a spear.

In other words, you first need the spear, or basic combat skills.

There are many people who possess a catalog of facts concerning certain aspects of the vital points, such as the "correct" time of day to strike a particular meridian for best results, the "correct" angle in which the points should be struck, the "correct" sequence in which these points should be struck, and so on. We shall see later just how useful or effective these aspects are, but none will be of any use whatsoever if the defender has no basic defensive techniques. However, the encouraging thing is that, after many years of research and actual hands-on experience (both personally and by the hundreds of law-enforcement officials and special-groups personnel throughout the world who use these techniques daily), I can tell you that it is not necessary to become involved in the minutiae of the use of kyusho jutsu. Much is ephemeral and most is unnecessary.

The use of the vital points to subdue an assailant is very important indeed and makes a tremendous difference in the effectiveness of defensive techniques. However, it takes some knowledge and a lot of practice. In this book I hope to show you a number of defensive tactics that—enhanced by the correct application of only a few vital points—will, without a doubt, make your techniques more powerful and much more effective.

The Mythology

You've inevitably read about or seen on the big screen an old kung fu master who uses mysterious martial skills from an ancient age, often wrapped in a philosophic pseudo-Zen ethic, to defeat bigger and stronger assailants. Legends of the "one-touch death" technique abound—even *Star Trek*'s Mr. Spock's Vulcan neck grip, which caused unconsciousness in an enemy, owes much to this mythic ability. Today we even have the nonsense of the "no-touch KO," which I will address later.

In truth, it is possible to kill an opponent with one blow, but it has nothing at all to do with some ancient mysterious knowledge (at one time, all knowledge was mysterious). One of the first recorded examples of striking vulnerable areas of the human body to bring about the defeat of an opponent occurs in *Nihongi*, an ancient Japanese work written or compiled around A.D. 720 which details an incident that took place in 23 B.C.

In it is a story concerning a powerful man named Kuyehaya, from the village of Taima, who boasted of his great strength. Hearing of this, the emperor summoned Nomi no Sukune from Idzumo to challenge him and test his claims that no one could stand against him. In the match that followed, they were made to wrestle against one another, but as they stood opposite each other, they both began using kicking techniques. Nomi no Sukune first broke Kuyehaya's ribs then kicked him in the loins and killed him. Although described as a wrestling match, this is perhaps the first recorded example of the use of *atemi-waza* ("striking techniques," here more correctly *ashi-ate*, "smashing with the foot or leg").

The human body is vulnerable to manipulation and attack in many ways, some demanding the application of great force, some requiring a lighter force. The effects on the body can be amplified by striking or manipulating certain areas rather than others. The determining factor is: What kind of effect do you want to produce?

Knockouts

First and foremost, the primary use of the vital points is *not* to cause unconsciousness but to facilitate all defensive techniques, which—in extreme circumstances—include those that render an attacker dizzy or unconscious. In any defensive situation, from the merely annoying right up to the defense of life itself, the vital points can improve the success of the defense. The cline of self-defense techniques is thus enhanced by the application of kyusho jutsu, the art of using the vital points.

Depending on the points used and the objective sought, a variety of effects can be produced. There are several degrees of what is known as a knockout:

- A transitory dizziness causing temporary physical lack of normal coordination.

- A longer period of dizziness and lack of coordination leading to the body's inability to maintain an upright position.

- A complete loss of consciousness for either a long or short period.

There are, of course, also degrees within these broad outlines.

Some points are more suitable for striking, others for applying pressure. Some points are best used in conjunction with others, while some can be attacked directly. In law enforcement, I teach officers to use vital points in order to gain and retain control of an uncooperative subject without causing more than minimal physical harm. With anti-terrorist and Special Forces squads, I escalate the training to the point of inducing unconsciousness. In civilian training, I concentrate primarily on escape and disabling methods.

The points are often used as non-striking aids when grappling and locking. However, one rule of thumb is never to grapple without striking first, even if only to startle and/or distract the attacker. As it is possible to inadvertently knock someone out by using the points, it is better to start with a brief look at the mechanism of the knockout. This will allow you to better understand the dangers of misuse and to promote safety in training.

The Causes

In broad terms, unconsciousness is brought about by stunning the brain or by starving it of blood (and therefore the oxygen that it needs in order to function). It is also possible to do both. A knockout, or loss of consciousness, can occur in three ways:

1. It can be induced by a severe blow to the head when the brain is injured as it bangs against the opposite side of the skull.

This type of knockout requires the stimulation of the upper spinal cord. The force of the blow must be at an angle that reaches and provokes a response in the basal ganglia. This in turn interrupts the reticular activating system (which is crucial for maintaining consciousness), disrupts motor function, and shuts down the brain.

2. It can be induced by causing a disruption in the blood flow to the brain.

This is inherently very dangerous as the longer the brain is starved of oxygenated blood, the greater the damage that occurs. For example, during a stroke, blood vessel blockage (which deprives the brain of blood, and thus oxygen) causes a loss of circulation to a part of the brain, thereby resulting in permanent loss of function.

Unconsciousness occurs after a short interval (generally between 12 and 20 seconds). Maintaining the disruption longer than this can lead to permanent damage and even death.

There are a number of ways in which this denial of oxygenated blood can be initiated. One method is to constrict the jugular vein and carotid artery in the neck. In combat terms, this is the basis of the lateral vascular choke hold, which blocks fresh, oxygenated blood from entering the brain while simultaneously preventing deoxygenated blood from flowing from the brain. The result is unconsciousness.

3. It can be induced by a sudden lowering of blood pressure.

It is also sometimes possible to induce a drop in blood pressure in the body to such a degree that dizziness and loss of consciousness occur. This is caused by the action of the baroreceptors. These are located in the walls of the arteries in the thorax as well as in the neck, and can be divided into high-pressure arterial baroreceptors and low-pressure baroreceptors. These detect the pressure of blood flowing through them, and can send messages to the central nervous system to increase or decrease blood pressure and heart rate. The baroreceptors will also report the information to the two areas of the medulla: the vasomotor center and the vagal center.

If, due to a strike or blow, arterial blood pressure increases, the firing rate of the baroreceptors increases, which sends a greater frequency of impulses to the brain. The reflex in this instance will cause stimulation of the vagus nerve, decreasing the heart rate in order to reduce arterial pressure. If the strike or blow is of a strength that does not cause any permanent damage to the underlying structure but is hard enough to activate the response from the baroreceptors, blood pressure decreases, thus reducing the firing and frequency of the baroreceptor signals. This activates the sympathetic nervous system, causing the heart to contract more rapidly and the blood vessels to constrict, to increase arterial blood pressure. Through this reflex circuit, the body's optimum arterial blood pressure is maintained.

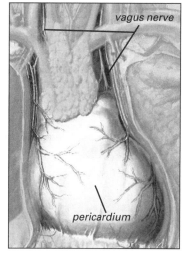

vagus nerve

pericardium

Note, however, that striking the vital points in order to manipulate the baroreceptors is not consistently reliable as the effects are markedly less in young, fit people. However, striking can be combined with pressure or constriction techniques for cumulative effects.

When the neck is struck or squeezed, it is possible to affect the vagus nerve, which starts in the brain and travels down into the abdomen. The vagus nerve is one of the most important nerves in the body, responsible for tasks such as heart rate, peristalsis, sweating, and several muscle movements in the mouth, including speech and keeping the larynx open for breathing. Stimulating the vagus nerve with a blow (commonly to the side of the neck, St.9, Li.17) will lead to a reduction in heart rate, blood pressure or both. If the degree of stimulation is sufficient, it will lead to a condition called vasovagal syncope. The most common symptoms of vasovagal syncope are dizziness and fainting; it occasionally leads to a complete loss of consciousness.

Techniques aimed at the neck might also adversely affect the phrenic nerve, which passes through the body and controls the movement of the diaphragm, and thus breathing. Damage to one side of the nerve is occasionally fatal, but usually leads to a dysfunction in one half of the diaphragm.

4. It can be induced by overstimulating and disrupting the central nervous system.

At the base of the brain is a small part of the brainstem called the reticular activating system (RAS). A disruption of the RAS may cause a person to pass out.

Physiological Factors

To understand the factors that bring about unconsciousness or dizziness (leaving aside the influence of drugs and/or hypnosis), it is necessary to have a basic grasp of human anatomy and physiology, especially if we wish to clear away the obfuscation and myth that often surround the subject in the martial arts. However tempting it may be, do not just flip to the "good bits"! Time spent learning anatomy and physiology will pay dividends in your training.

In a straightforward KO (i.e., non–"vital point"—actually a misnomer, but more on this later), a force of impact at the front of the head, be it from a punch or a blow from any hard object, causes the brain to crash against the hard bone of the skull that encases it. This is a dual impact—at the front initially, then at the rear—and these impacts, if severe enough, cause a neurological reaction in the area of the brain near the back of the skull. This reaction serves as a protective mechanism and shuts down brain activity.

Part of this defensive reaction is due to interference with the normal activity of the basal ganglia, which work together with the cerebellum to help control normal physical activity. The motor cortex sends information to both the ganglia and the cerebellum, and both structures send information straight to the cortex, passing through the thalamus. The basic function of the nervous responses of the cerebellum is to excite the system, while that of the basal ganglia is to decrease activity in the system. The balance between these two functions promotes smooth, coordinated movement, and any imbalance or disruption in either will create movement dysfunction.

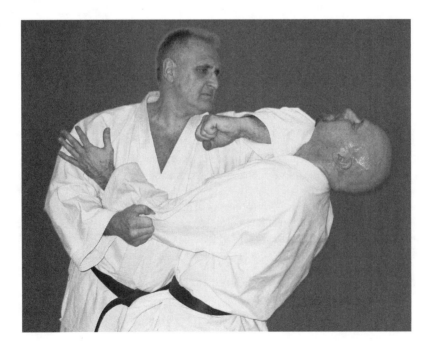

Pressure Point Physiology

Kyusho jutsu is not just the art of rendering an opponent unconscious, which is often inappropriate. It also serves to manipulate the body's responses in a predictable manner, which facilitates effective defensive combat techniques. Knowing basic anatomy and physiology is essential to understanding how pressure points work. This section covers the more pertinent functions of the organs that are manipulated in kyusho jutsu.

Amygdala

The amygdala, a remnant of the oldest part of the brain structure, helps process emotions such as fear and aggression; triggers the sympathetic nervous system; and is responsible for initiating the "fight or flight" response and muscular reflex actions such as the withdrawal response. In terms of combat, this is a very important organ in that it is responsible for triggering reflexive reactions to stimuli that cannot be overridden by the cerebral cortex's commands to stop the reflex action.

Assuming that the stimulus is unexpected, the actions of the amygdala and the cortex are roughly simultaneous, but the amygdala has priority. Thus a withdrawal reaction to a painful stimulus will always take priority over the conscious command to dismiss the stimulus as unimportant or non-threatening. If, however, the brain has received early warning, the cortex can initiate a response in advance to ignore the reflex command. In some cases, this has some effect.

Reticular Activating System

The human body, in every living moment, maintains a number of automatic functions such as breathing, maintaining appropriate heart rate and blood pressure, and ensuring correct muscle activity for correct balance and movement. While some of this is under a degree of conscious control, in general the reticular activating system

(RAS) works quietly in the background of everyday life and is largely undetected and unappreciated; it is a kind of automatic pilot. Disruption of the RAS can affect the level of consciousness and can even lead to unconsciousness and coma. Physically, the RAS is a network of nerves that extend from the lower brainstem into the pons, midbrain, thalamus and cerebral cortex.

Basal Ganglia and Cerebellum

The basal ganglia and cerebellum are large collections of nuclei that modify movement on a minute-to-minute basis. The motor cortex sends information to both, and both structures transmit information right back to the cortex via the thalamus. Disrupting the balance between the excitatory and inhibitory brain systems (the basal ganglia being inhibitory and the cerebellum being excitatory) will cause a loss in the ability to maintain coordinated movement and posture. This is significant in that it can affect the reactions of an assailant's body, to the advantage of an expert defender, by provoking an inappropriate response.

The cerebellum, for the most part, coordinates movement by maintaining the balance between antagonistic muscle groups, especially in times of rapid movement and changes in position. The cerebellum compares what actually happens with what was expected to happen and is capable of making corrections and adjustments. In martial arts terms, any strike or manipulation that causes a disruption in the main function of the cerebellum is advantageous. For example, an elbow strike to Gb.20 on the back of the neck will cause major disruption to the RAS and to the activity of the cerebellum.

Brainstem

The brainstem (midline or middle of brain) includes the midbrain, the pons, and the medulla. Functions of this area include movement of the eyes and mouth, relaying sensory messages (hot, pain, loud), hunger, respiration, consciousness, cardiac function, blood pressure, body temperature, involuntary muscle movements, sneezing, coughing, vomiting and swallowing. The brainstem also serves to maintain an upright posture. Any blow or stimulus powerful enough to disrupt brainstem function will certainly cause loss of balance and can have an adverse effect on cardiac function and consciousness.

The Autonomic Nervous System

The autonomic nervous system (ANS), the supervisory system of the body's internal environment, is divided into the sympathetic and the parasympathetic systems. Under the supervision of the hypothalamus and the brainstem, the ANS controls heart rate, blood vessel constriction, the digestive system and much more. It is not normally under conscious control.

The sympathetic system is responsible, among a host of other tasks, for reacting to stress by releasing noradrenaline into the circulatory system; the sympathetic response has often been described as preparation for "fight or flight." When this system is activated, it affects the whole body rather than individual organs, with the result that heart and metabolic rates are increased to help cope with an emergency situation. The process of digestion is temporarily halted and blood vessels near the surface of the skin constrict while blood flow to major organs is enhanced. The pupils of the eyes dilate in order to better perceive movement and the whole body is geared up to act in an optimum fashion.

The parasympathetic system is concerned with the regular and normal functions of the body, e.g., changing food into energy and eliminating waste material. It complements the actions of the sympathetic nervous system, such as decreasing heart rate and blood pressure when the sympathetic response has increased both.

The Use of Reflexive Responses
in Self-Defense

Fighter pilots in dogfights routinely learn the same skill as the expert game hunter, which is never to aim directly at your target, but ahead of it so that the missile/bullet/shotgun pellets arrive simultaneously with the target at a predicted place in space and time. In any physical combat, knowing in advance where your target will be is an obvious advantage. To be able to ensure that the opponent always goes to the predicted place, regardless of his intentions, is again another obvious advantage.

The human body has a number of vulnerable areas that, if correctly struck or manipulated, will force the opponent into just such a predictable position. This therefore allows the counterstrike or technique to be delivered much more quickly than if one had to wait to see what the opponent's reaction would be. When pressure is applied, the nerves send a message to the spine. From here, the message is directed straight back to the affected organ, which will simultaneously initiate the response as it sends a signal to the brain.

Note that the body does not wait for the brain to decide on the degree of danger in the message—it could be too late to stop damage from occurring. Therefore the reflex action moves the organ away from the potential danger, just in case. For example, the fleshy underarm skin just above and to the inside of the triceps muscle can be pinched and twisted sharply to force a rapid withdrawal of the arm. This is a technique we teach for dealing with low-level nuisance assaults and to children to ward off a bully without causing any harm. The fast onset of sharp pain invokes an involuntary snatching away of the arm from the source of the pain. Other areas of the body, such as the nipples and the insides of the thighs, are also particularly sensitive to this type of defense.

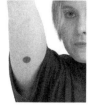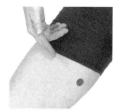

A sample of pinch areas.

The Flinch Reflex

The flinch (flexion) reflex, also known as the withdrawal reflex, responds to potentially damaging stimuli, such as placing a hand on a hot stove or stepping on a sharp object. In such an instance, a rapid withdrawal response is invoked to protect from damage.

One of the most important features of this reflexive response is that it is accompanied by what is known as a crossed-extension reflex action. If, for example, you were to step with your bare foot on a sharp pebble, this extension reflex action would automatically brace the muscles in the other leg in order to maintain balance while rapidly withdrawing the leg in danger. Keeping this in mind, we know that when we strike or manipulate one of an attacker's arms, we can force the other arm to reflexively move out to the side and be unable to help the attacker.

The Stretch and Inverse Stretch Reflex

All muscles have mechanisms that detect changes in muscle tension brought about by stretch actions, which may be active or passive. The stretch, or myotatic, reflex, responds to passive stretching and is an important element in the automatic maintenance of posture and muscle tone. The reaction causes an automatic tightening of the muscle to avoid overstretching or tearing. The inverse stretch reflex, also known as the Golgi tendon reflex, reacts to muscle tension by relaxing the muscle again to avoid structural damage.

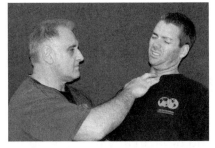

Triggering the gag reflex.

This latter reaction is extremely useful in combat, and especially so in the application of armlocks and strikes to the arms or legs to force the body to move into a vulnerable position. The value of these reactions lies in the fact that they do not depend upon great physical strength, but upon accuracy of technique.

The Gag Reflex

The gag reflex can be invoked by jabbing the fingertips sharply into the throat just above the sternal notch. It can be designated as Conception Vessel 22, but here the point is used as a label only, as the withdrawal reflex owes nothing to any Chinese medical implications but to the urgent reflexive command to move away from perceived danger. The angle should be slightly upwards, and the motion must be fast. Initially there may be a reaction to the pain, but it is the gag reflex—not the pain factor—that compels the body to move away from the strike.

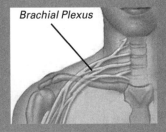

Brachial Plexus

The Brachial Plexus

Correctly angled blows to the junction of the shoulder and neck can deliver a temporarily disorientating shock that can stun the brain and affect the use of the arm. This is a popular technique in some law-enforcement training as there is minimal risk to the assailant, and is preferable to other strikes that could inflict damage. It also does not give rise to an adrenaline rush, therefore the assailant is unlikely to increase the level of his resistance or assault.

Startle Reflex

Sometimes movement without any touch at all can be used to bring about a reflex action, as anyone who has ever glimpsed something out of the corner of their eye moving rapidly and unexpectedly towards them will have experienced—they've probably reflexively ducked and raised their hands in a protective flinch. Remember that using only a reflexive point will not normally be enough to end a determined attack. What it will do is end the immediate threat to the defender and allow the opportunity to either escape or to deliver the coup de grâce, so to speak, of a disabling strike or a control hold.

Keep in mind that the invocation should be fast, and/or unexpected. A slow movement towards the groin or face will not trigger the startle reflex, and a slow application of pressure will not generate the sudden withdrawal reflex.

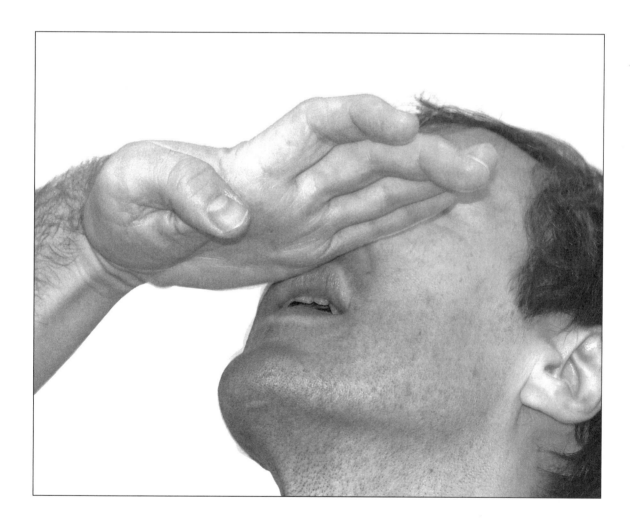

The Traditional Significance
of Ki or Chi

Chinese tradition maintains the view that the whole universe is filled with and permeated by a "vital force" or source of power that they call *chi* (also spelled *qi*; it's *ki* in Japanese). In ages past, it was thought possible that by developing and manipulating this force, one could attain immortality, and through specialized training one could become impervious to harm in combat. According to the ancient Taoist scripture *Great Peace Extensive Record*, "One who has become immortal is immune from all calamity. Heaven and Earth might be engulfed and still he would remain unscathed: how much less could he be injured by ordinary weapons?"

By utilizing special breathing and training techniques, the belief was that chi could strengthen not just the internal organs but even the bones, too. Unfortunately, researching the written records of early examples promoting the benefits accrued from practicing these special arts only causes one to raise an eyebrow in disbelief.

In the preface to the 1881 edition of the *I Chin Ching*, editor Wang Tsu-Yuan related his own experience as a young and weak youth. He stated that at the age of 13, he was taught the exercises by a military officer, and that after one year he felt very healthy. His strength was so developed that he could lift "the accumulated weight of ten *chuan*."

All well and good, except that ten *chuan* was the equivalent of about 400 pounds! To believe that any 14-year-old could out-lift the huge, muscle-laden participants in the world's strongest man event is beyond belief.

However, to return to the origins of these beliefs: The milieu which brought them about was the same one that discouraged the dissection of bodies to accurately discover the internal structures of the organs of the human body. Thus Chinese medicine had little understanding of how the internal organs actually worked, and had only a hazy comprehension of blood circulation. Nonetheless, there arose a concept that all of the vital organs of the human body were connected via an invisible and intangible series of conduits called "meridians," along which chi—the invisible and intangible "life force," or energy—traveled, nourishing the body when kept in balance.

Martial schools adopted these beliefs and designed patterns of exercises to promote the "balance" of the internal organs while strengthening them for combat. In an age of spirits and demons, where—as today—knowledge is power, the unscrupulous were always ready to take advantage of the unwary. A school purporting to teach the ability to kill or maim at a distance, or with the slightest of touches, was obviously going to be more popular than any that rested its laurels upon the purely physical and mechanical.

To begin to understand the strength of such beliefs, even centuries after their inception, one only has to remember the experiences of the Chinese in the Boxer Rebellion (1898). They believed that through their martial training they were impervious to bullets. Unfortunately, they died in the thousands.

Sadly, even today there are some martial artists who feel the need to "tap into" a mysterious, extraordinary force to enhance their prowess and their health. A casual online search will immediately generate hundreds of sites offering courses that will purportedly give the reader the power to manipulate chi through a series of exercise and meditation programs. The claims by many are outrageous: "Move objects with Chi Power without touching them." "Move an object with your eyes only." "Extinguish a candle flame with your eyes only." "For speed faster than a cat, try this test." "Lift a bowl of water with Yin Chi." "Learn how to make select breaks." "Ring the chimes with a Yang Chi throw." "Repel birds, dogs, with your eyes only."

In Evan Pantazi's modern book about pressure point fighting, the author propagates the erroneous information that striking points will "stop most of the energy from reaching the organs and thus cause their failure." Although I do believe that (to quote *Hamlet*) "there are more things in heaven and earth, Horatio, Than are dreamt of in your philosophy," to perpetuate the myth that there is a mysterious energy which acts upon individual organs of the body and can be used in combat is, frankly, unacceptable in light of modern medical knowledge.

It should not be assumed that the Chinese belief in a mystical life force is or was somehow unique. Far from it! The ancient Greeks following Aristotle held a similar belief in the theory of the four humors, which stated that the body is composed of a balance between the four elements present on earth: fire, earth, water and air. These were manifested in the body as yellow bile, black bile, blood and phlegm.

In medieval Europe, the work of the second-century doctor Galen served to spread the idea that the health of every human being was controlled by a balance of four bodily fluids: blood, yellow bile, black bile and phlegm, called the "humors." It was an imbalance of these humors, Galen said, that lay at the bottom of every illness, and good health could be restored by regaining the correct balance. The methods of treatment included bleeding a patient until this was achieved.

In Elizabethan Europe, medical belief was heavily influenced by this theory of humors. Today, we can see a remnant of this belief in our use of the term "melancholy," which comes from the Greek for "black bile," an overabundance of which was thought to lead to despondency and depression. Later medical discoveries in Europe eventually led to the complete abandonment of these archaic beliefs, but as such experimentation was frowned upon in China, the transition from philosophical belief to a modern medical system was expectedly far slower.

In modern times, Kirlian photography, which purported to capture on film the "bio-plasmic" energy emanating from all living things, was thought to prove the existence of the life force. In the end, however, it turned out that the photographs were capturing an aura that was recording the degree of moisture present, with nothing at all to do with any mysterious "force." Once again, I must reiterate that there is no scientific or medical proof whatsoever of the existence of this "force."

Debunking Tradition

Given that early Chinese doctors and martial artists had little or only rudimentary knowledge of the workings of the internal organs of the human body, it is not surprising that they developed an empirical approach to both healing and disrupting the balance of the body. The theory of acupuncture (and its ally acupressure, or shiatsu) is that the human body contains several conduits, or meridians, which connect the vital organs and act as channels for the movement of chi.

To date there is no scientifically accepted evidence that can verify the anatomical or histological existence of acupuncture points or meridians. Proponents of traditional Chinese medicine claim that it is a prescientific system that nevertheless continues to be effective today.

Just as with chi, no one has ever been able to show or prove the existence of these meridians in circulatory, nervous or lymphatic systems. The best scientific research has, however, indicated that acupuncture does have some analgesic effect in some circumstances. In other words, it can have a limited pain-relief effect. It is not, however, the panacea that its proponents would claim.

There is still controversy and the debate continues. The National Institutes for Health concludes: "Acupuncture as a therapeutic intervention is widely practiced in the United States. While there have been many studies of its potential usefulness, many of these studies provide equivocal results because of design, sample size, and other factors. The issue is further complicated by inherent difficulties in the use of appropriate controls, such as placebos and sham acupuncture groups. However, promising results have emerged, for example, showing efficacy of acupuncture in adult postoperative and chemotherapy nausea and vomiting and in postoperative dental pain. There are other situations, such as addiction, stroke rehabilitation, headache, menstrual cramps, tennis elbow, fibromyalgia, myofascial pain, osteoarthritis, low back pain, carpal tunnel syndrome, and asthma, in which acupuncture may be useful as an adjunct treatment or an acceptable alternative or be included in a comprehensive management program. Further research is likely to uncover additional areas where acupuncture interventions will be useful."

The American Medical Association, on the other hand, adopted the following statement as policy in 1997 after assessing a number of alternative therapies, including acupuncture: "There is little evidence to confirm the safety or efficacy of most alternative therapies. Much of the information currently known about these therapies makes it clear that many have not been shown to be efficacious. Well-designed, stringently controlled research should be done to evaluate the efficacy of alternative therapies."

In 1995, the Committee for the Scientific Investigation of Claims of the Paranormal (CSICOP) sent a party to China to investigate a number of claims being made by qigong (or *chi gung*) masters and their young students, who "supposedly possessed what Chinese admirers call 'special ability' or 'extraordinary functions of the human body.'" They were said to be able to alter the shape or color of objects in sealed containers and perform a host of other minor miracles. The first CSICOP delegation (composed of most of the executive council at the time) found that these children could not produce their effects under close observation. In short, the whiz kids and their masters were performing unsophisticated conjuring tricks (Alcock et al. 1988). Also, in controlled tests, the delegation found the vaunted abilities of the qigong masters to diagnose medical ailments to be "unsubstantiated."

Following President Richard Nixon's visit to China in 1972, many of the Western journalists who accompanied him, and many of the doctors who followed later, were subject to much propaganda on behalf of the traditional Chinese medical establishment. They were shown major surgery being performed with only acupuncture being used as an anesthetic. For example, columnist James Reston required an emergency appendectomy during Nixon's visit, and he was widely, though wrongly, believed to have received only acupuncture as a pain killer during the surgery. It was not until much later that it was revealed that the Chinese surgical patients observed by foreign delegations had been pre-selected for high pain tolerance and heavily indoctrinated beforehand. It was also disclosed that these demonstration cases were routinely given surreptitious doses of morphine in an intravenous drip that supposedly contained only hydrating and nourishing fluids (Keng and Tao 1985). In addition, it has since come to light that much of the apparently objective and well-controlled research on traditional Chinese medicine emanating from Chinese medical schools during the upheaval of the cultural revolution (1966–1976) was falsified at the behest of the hospitals' scientifically unqualified political commissars to ensure that the "research" would support the party line.

Despite this prevarication, through further visits and investigations, most experts today concede that acupuncture does have some analgesic properties, though its potency has been greatly exaggerated. The bulk of these effects, however, can be explained in modern Western medical terms by the effect of endorphins and other analgesic secretions produced by the body in response to the "treatment." One explanation of the effects produced is the "pain gate" theory, which concludes that acupuncture's anesthetic results are brought about by the stimulation of the nerves by the needles, which serve to block the passage of stronger pain impulses along the same nerve, and thus deaden the pain.

As for the existence of conduits or "meridians," Felix Mann, founder and past president of the Medical Acupuncture Society, the first president of the British Medical Acupuncture Society, and the author of

The Five-Element Cycle Theory

In brief, the five-element cycle appears to be a later addition to the corpus of Chinese medicine and it propounds that using acupuncture points in a specific order can have either a beneficial or a detrimental effect on the human body. The use of this cycle to select appropriate combinations of kyusho points to strike in order to enhance the effects of a technique is simply incorrect, even by Chinese medicine terms. Advocates of the theory maintain that as there is a cycle of construction in acupuncture, so there is a valid cycle of destruction.

Essentially, in the Chinese medical system, the body's organs are kept in a healthy balance by the unrestricted flow of chi through a number of meridians that connect them. The two universal forces of yin and yang (negative and positive), when in balance, promote a healthy body. Any disturbance of this balance could be provoked by either overloading an organ with the flow of chi, or by blocking the flow. Manipulating various corresponding points on the affected meridians, by heat, pressure or needle, would set the system in balance again.

As the constructive cycle was determined to have beneficial effects, so it was posited that there existed its mirror image, so to speak, which would negatively affect the harmonious balance of chi, and therefore weaken the body. Thus, in combat, to add to effects of a blow one should follow the latter sequence: Fire, Metal, Wood, Earth and Water.

There are a number of objections to this. In any physical confrontation, you take what you are given; there is no time to consider which combination of points you will be aiming for. The whole concept is further plunged into the realms of the ridiculous if you add to the equation that to get the best effect, you should strike points on different meridians at different times of the day. Another factor to consider is that in Chinese medicine, the original use of the five-element cycle theory was restricted to points on the limbs, and then only to those at or around the elbow or knee joint and lower down towards the extremities. This fact has been selectively overlooked by many proponents of this theory who have gone on to apply it to the whole body.

The five-element cycle:
exterior, constructive, interior, destructive

In 1999 at the University of Sussex in England, Mike Flanagan, a shiatsu student who attended many of my training sessions in the U.K., helped another martial artist, Zoltan Dienes, Ph.D., set up an experiment determining whether or not the use of any particular sequence of strikes showed any statistical benefit. Although the study was fairly small (28 participants), it did demonstrate that, as perceived by the subjects, there was no benefit accrued from the use of the destructive cycle in terms of the level of pain inflicted.

In my decades of experience, I fully agree that applying techniques in conjunction with each other can be beneficial, but this is to either invoke an involuntary reflex that can then be used to the defender's advantage, or to overload the system with pain. Never have I found it necessary to spend any time considering either the time of day or the striking sequence in terms of the five-element cycle theory.

Reinventing Acupuncture: A New Concept of Ancient Medicine, states that "traditional acupuncture points are no more real than the black spots a drunkard sees in front of his eyes" and "the meridians of acupuncture are no more real than the meridians of geography. If someone were to get a spade and tried to dig up the Greenwich meridian, he might end up in a lunatic asylum. Perhaps the same fate should await those doctors who believe in meridians."

The human body can be made to react in predictable ways by stimulating special locations that are peculiarly responsive to stimuli. It is possible to create a flinch reaction, a momentary physical imbalance, a loss of motor function, dizziness and even total loss of consciousness and death by methods that are well explained by human physiology. There is no need whatsoever to resort to archaic mysticism. The use of the vital points is so important that all irrelevant and misleading pseudo-science should be stripped away and the truth—that they are of paramount importance in self-defense systems—recognized and accepted.

The Dichotomy

Knowledge of the use of vital points handed down over the ages has been, out of necessity, transcribed in terms of this Chinese medical system, and has ascribed the effects produced by the manipulation of these vital points to the action of chi either being denied to the organ or overwhelming it. It would be remiss to dismiss the use of the system of denoting the points by their acupuncture nomenclature since this "road map" of where the points are situated is very useful if understood. Consider it something akin to a circuit diagram of an electrical system, for instance, or knowing where the light switches are in a building. It isn't necessary to understand electromagnetic theory nor building construction if you just need to turn on the light. You only need to know where the switches are.

Therefore, this book presents the most important kyusho points on diagrams following the pattern of acupuncture charts, which retain conventional acupuncture labeling.

Regarding the point known as Lu.5, the actual position for optimum results is not actually on the acupuncture point at all. The so-called Lu.5 strike is in fact delivered approximately one inch below the Chinese medicine designated point. Again, a major law-enforcement training group originally taught the officers to apply pressure to the actual Tw.17 site. This did indeed generate a degree of pain; however, for the very best results it is necessary to insert the thumbs directly behind the ear lobes high up at the back of the jaw, thus affecting the fifth facial nerve. The technique should be done sharply in an inward and upward direction with a vibrating motion of the thumbs. The pain is excruciating and has the charac urn away and move both hands to his ears.

The Kyusho (Vital) Points

The use of the vital points has definite advantages. It's relatively easy to learn and apply, which is important for non–martial artists interested in learning self-defense techniques and for law-enforcement agents who may not have any martial background. Frankly, if your main concern is to develop defensive skills, it is often better not to be a martial artist steeped in the regular practice of sports techniques (which, by definition, are crafted to be not dangerous). However, for martial artists, the addition (or, rather, the re-introduction) of the use of vital points to a neutered sports-oriented system gives greater depth to the system and makes the defensive *waza* ("techniques") much more effective.

Legally, the use of the vital points allows the subduing and control of a combative subject with none of the external physical trauma that would be expected from generalized, non-point-specific strikes to the head, face or torso. It is therefore inherently more legally defensible, as it demonstrates the desire to uphold the safety of the aggressor as much as is possible. The results of vital point strikes—either to stun or to cause motor dysfunction—are negligible or produce only minor bruising.

The basic kyusho techniques can be applied under high levels of stress and do not depend upon fine motor control, which deteriorates markedly under stress. The practice of these techniques can also be carried out in comparative safety, allowing a high number of repetitions to "groove" the required response into the defender. Remember, without constant practice of correct tactics and the basics, knowledge of the vital points is of limited usefulness.

In critical self-defense situations, it is best to use a technique that will induce a shockwave type of effect and create a neurological shutdown, however briefly. These techniques require only one point to be struck. In a lower-level situation, such as in an arrest and control procedure, it is possible to escalate simple control techniques to a knockout by using more than one point strike; the accumulation of pain stimuli arriving at the brain simultaneously causes a shutdown. This needs to be done very quickly, moving from the limbs up towards the head. The effectiveness of this type of technique depends on generating significant pain very rapidly at a small number (conventionally three) of points to cause overload in the receptors, which react in order to protect the brain from this sudden, shocking attack.

It is better *not* to practice many techniques—fewer is better in self-defense. It is a well-documented physiological fact that under great stress, the mind is unable to choose between a variety of techniques. Selecting a technique can be done when the first shock is survived. It is far better to have one technique that will operate successfully in a number of different attack scenarios than to learn a different technique for each one.

Martial artists wishing to consult earlier recorded sources regarding the location and use of the vital points will find that there is a distinct difference between the charts and usage theories from Japan (via Okinawa) and those of China, especially when linking points in order to enhance the effectiveness of a technique.

This section covers the locations of some of the more useful vital points used in the application of vital-point kyusho techniques. The traditional Chinese terminology is also shown for reference. Some indication is given of the manner in which the points are used, and the weapons with which the results are brought about.

Keep in mind that this is only an introduction to the most useful points, not an exhaustive treatise. This information will, however, allow you to maximize the effects of your defense skills. You do not have to memorize every point—your technique will guide you to the correct response and target area; knowledge of the points often simply explains why a technique works. Nothing will take the place of direct instruction, so diligent readers should seek out a competent teacher to progress their knowledge.

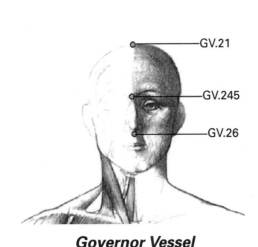

GV.21

GV.245

GV.26

CV.24

CV.22

CV.17

CV.14

CV.8

CV.4

Governor Vessel   **Conception Vessel**

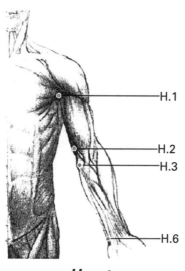

Heart

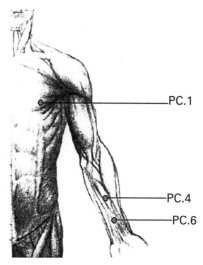

Pericardium

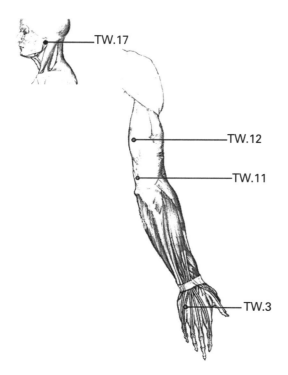

Triple Warmer

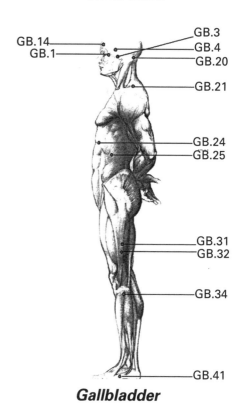

Gallbladder

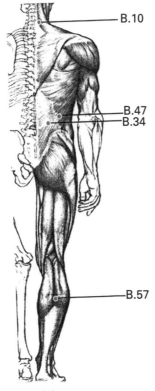

— B.10

— B.47
— B.34

— B.57

Bladder

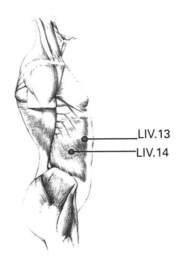

— LIV.13
— LIV.14

Liver

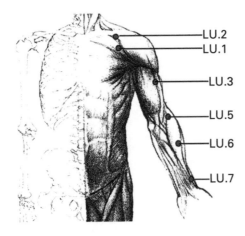

— LU.2
— LU.1

— LU.3

— LU.5

— LU.6

— LU.7

Lung

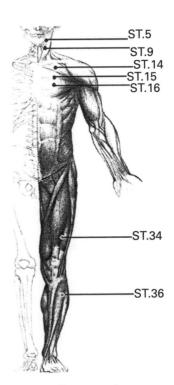

— ST.5
— ST.9
— ST.14
— ST.15
— ST.16

— ST.34

— ST.36

Stomach

THE SECRET ART OF PRESSURE POINT FIGHTING

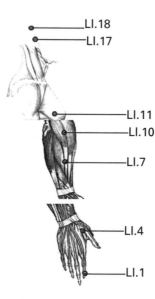

Large Intestine

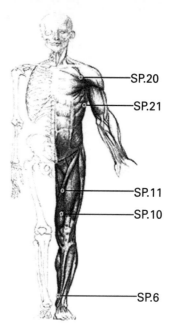

Spleen

The Kyusho Weapons

Any part of the body can be used as a weapon, the most common ones being the head, fist, straight fingers, palm heel, elbows, knees and feet.

Inside/outside defenses

When attacked with a strike, it is inherently safer to move to the outside of whichever arm the attacker uses to initiate the assault. This position makes it very challenging for him to use his other arm, thus effectively disposing of one of his major weapons. The position of his body in relation to yours will also make it extremely difficult for him to kick you. In addition to being safer for the defendant, moving to the outside gives easy access to some of the major knockdown points and control techniques. This is frequently a method of choice in law enforcement when subduing and handcuffing a struggling perpetrator.

In instances where tables, chairs, people, and other barriers make it impossible for you to move the outside position, it is possible to move inside, or into the opponent's space. This can be advantageous because, since it will be totally unexpected, you gain easy access to a number of vital points, which can end the fight abruptly. The only proviso is that you must act very quickly to obtain and retain the advantage.

Roundhouse block

No matter what type of attack the assailant makes with his hands, be it a punch, a push or a grab, it is always beneficial to use the roundhouse block. This is a technique seen frequently in karate kata (solo practice form), but unfortunately little used in practice. It does, however, form the basis of an effective defensive move to either the inside or the outside position and gives the defender great opportunity to deflect, seize and control the attacking limb in order to bring about a knockdown or control.

At first glance, the roundhouse block appears to be a complicated maneuver, yet children ages five or six can perform this competently after only a few training sessions. It is well worth persisting with and actually is the basis of every other blocking movement in karate.

The optimum hand position (open, facing the attacker in an apparent defensive, non-threatening position) is ideal for performing this roundhouse block.

The attacking hand or fist is first deflected by the open palm of what is generally considered to be the attacking or rear hand, which moves in a circular movement over the other leading (front) hand.

This takes the initial power of the blow away from the target and positions the attacker's arm for the following strike or further deflection to injure the limb and unbalance the assailant.

Frisbee block

In situations where an attacker throws his strongest punch or attempts to strike with a club, by far most effective defense is what we in Kissaki-Kai karate call the "frisbee block." The objective is to use the defender's extended arm to jam the attacker's arm before it develops full momentum. This is done by thrusting the arm as if throwing a frisbee past the attacker's head so that the forearm of the assailant smacks into the defender's extended forearm just below the elbow. Because of the anatomy of the arm, this will cause the attacker's Pc.6 or Lu.5 point to impact the defender's arm with great force, thus disabling the attacker's arm and making him unable to use it in a further attack.

A further benefit of the frisbee block is that it places the defender's blocking arm in a perfect position to continue the defense by striking the assailant's neck and head. It also places the defender inside the attacker's arms in the ideal position to deliver a headbutt attack to the attacker's face—an altogether excellent defensive position.

frisbee block

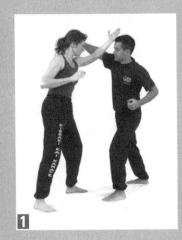
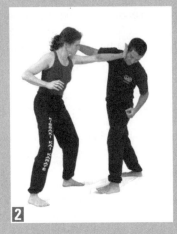
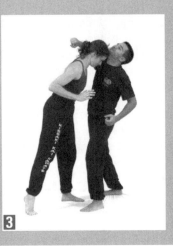

**mawashi uke
(roundhouse block)**

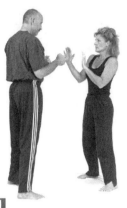

1

Optimum hand position for performing a roundhouse block.

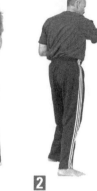

2

Open palm first deflects the attacking fist, circling over the defender's front hand.

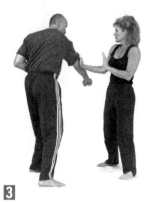

3

Further deflection with front hand.

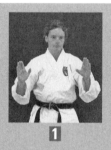

1

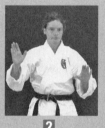

2

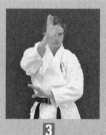

3

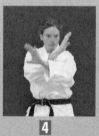

4

**mawashi uke
(roundhouse block)**

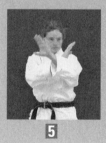

5

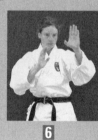

6

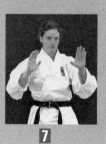

7

Stimulating the Pressure Points

Pinching and twisting the skin has a long tradition in the Chinese art of Chin Na, and many of the Okinawa karate masters were famed for having a grip so strong that they could strip the bark from trees and crush bamboo. Before I studied the martial arts in depth, I had assumed that the development of a strong grip was simply to aid in the execution of throwing techniques. My research soon revealed, however, that pinching and twisting the skin in vulnerable areas of the human body can introduce severe and sudden pain and a consequential withdrawal reflex. Pinches make great distraction techniques that momentarily confuse an attacker and break his concentration long enough for a more conclusive defensive technique to be executed.

As with modern karate, modern ju-jutsu also lost some of its original effective defensive techniques (*waza*) from its repertoire. Pinching and twisting the skin are two of these.

"The 'pinches' to which reference is so often made are not only no longer used, but are not even permitted in any Ju-Jutsu contest at any of the important meetings held in Japan. I am afraid that any man who depended on one of these 'pinches' in order to secure a victory in a serious contest would find himself sadly disappointed. These 'pinches' are absolutely banned together with hitting, finger gripping and twisting or using the hand on an opponent's face."

> *The Text Book of Ju-Jutsu as Practiced in Japan*
> S. K. Uyenishi, 1918. Pp. 18-19

Unlike simply pinching the skin in order to evoke a reflex response, another method is to push sharply into a vital point with the thumb joint or finger knuckle joint. However, this must be done with a vibrating action so that the pressure is continually increased and decreased, so that the system never has a chance to become used to the pain. Grabbing, twisting, pinching and applying pressure as above has a long tradition in the Oriental martial arts, forming a large part of Chin Na (trapping and controlling) repertoire. To facilitate their skills in this area, many of the old masters would condition their hands and fingers by continually striking them against a straw-covered post (*makiwara*); some even gained a reputation for being able to rend the bark from trees with the strength of their grip.

Rules of Combat and Awareness

Battles, either between individuals or nations, are instigated by men and fought by men. They are never indefinable or ad hoc in nature; they have always proceeded in discernible patterns from which it is possible to determine sets of rules—rules that can later be studied and from which sets of tactical procedures can be formulated. This truism forms the basis of all military tactical thinking.

If this supposition is correct, and if these "rules of combat" exist, how might they be helpful to a martial artist or anyone attempting to further their understanding and expertise in the areas of the martial arts or self-defense? These rules have indeed existed since warriors came into being and man's combative history was recorded. They can be studied and utilized by a warrior to gain an advantage in forthcoming encounters.

Colonel Rex Applegate, who functioned as Franklin D. Roosevelt's bodyguard, served in Military Intelligence and the Counter Intelligence Corps during World War II and was in charge of special close-combat training. He stated that there are a number of fundamental principles in hand-to-hand combat, from those that must be observed at all times to others that are only used in special circumstances. Only the user can determine which one is being utilized at a specific point in time. "Military experience…has shown that the average man can quickly be turned into a dangerous, offensive fighter by concentrating on a few basic principles of combat and by advocating principally the use of blows executed by the hands, feet and other parts of the body."

Consider a street attack, a sexual assault, and a terrorist bloodbath. Surely these are moments of such utter madness and fear that they are, by their very nature, beyond all understanding and all "rules"? The answer, fortunately, is no. Violent and sudden as these terrifying occasions might be, they work according to fairly well-defined sets of rules. By understanding these rules, it may be possible to survive such situations and to some extent understand both their mechanics and the evolving pressures that produce them.

However, it is impossible to consider this subject by confining it only to those "rules" that appertain to the immediate physical safety of the defender in any personal physical confrontation, as there are other major influencing factors with their own particular sets of rules which have a defining or limiting effect upon this. Here I refer to the sets of values (cultural, religious, ethical) inherent in any society at any one particular moment and, in addition, the regulation of combat decided upon, imposed on and conditioned by the current militaristic or pacifistic ethos. These factors have an enormous influence upon the actual methods of combat, both personal and national (i.e., in civilian self-defense and in military operations), and play a role in determining what is acceptable or not acceptable, legal or illegal.

Rules of how to physically act in the stress of combat in order to save one's own life (or indeed that of others) or gain safety cannot be divorced from the possibility of legal consequences if a panel of jurors decides later that your response was not legally justifiable. Times and mores change. What is morally and legally acceptable on the battlefield may well be indefensible in a nightclub. It is important to be aware of the ramifications of applying indiscriminate defensive techniques. They may well save the situation, but perhaps better chosen methods would achieve the same result without the prospect of litigation.

Simply stated, in most civilized societies it is considered quite acceptable to use physical force to stop someone from attacking you, but you cannot hurt him too much, and as soon as he indicates that he has finished attacking you it becomes illegal for you to make sure he cannot do so again by continuing to strike him. This is now retaliation, not self-defense.

In essence, there are technical, practical ways in which an individual can defend himself or herself from an attacker. There are also ways in which external influences (cultural, ethical, legal) impinge upon these physical actions to the extent that the victim's ability to carry out a successful defense could be detrimentally affected. Luckily, by making use of the vulnerable areas of the body (the vital points), it is possible to halt and disable an attacker without resorting to simple, bludgeoning brute-force methods that may be interpreted later as overly violent. By adding the Rules of Combat into the equation, the odds of surviving an assault both physically and legally are vastly enhanced.

First, let's deal with a commonplace reaction: How can such apparently chaotic things as fights possibly have any rules? After all, aren't they all different, and don't they range in degrees of danger, from the potentially lethal (utilizing weapons) to simple, unarmed altercations? Surely you cannot have "rules" for all these and the many other possibilities or manifestations of personal combat?

Simply put, "Yes, you can!"

Most people (except those in the field of law enforcement) rarely experience more than, at an unlucky worst, just a few of these different possibilities, but they can draw together and study the various sources of evidence from both contemporary and historical sources. In doing so, certain common elements soon become apparent and it is indeed possible to deduce specific rules that can be used to gain an advantage in these situations. Military handbooks, for example, are based entirely upon the supposition that it is possible to set down a series of procedures that will enhance the effectiveness and safety of their soldiers to the detriment of the enemy. That this has always been the case can be judged from the long ancestry of these, one of the earliest being recorded in the Han History Bibliographies, which was completed around the year 90 B.C. This collection of chapters dealt with combative military skills to promote a greater efficiency in future battles.

In brief, if you are determined to develop and practice a system of defensive techniques that will be effective in the vast majority of situations, then you *must* learn the correct use of the vital points to weaken the attacker, and the tactical rules that will offer you optimum conditions in which to carry out the techniques.

Some of the Rules of Combat

1. Achieve *mushin*—literally "no mind." This refers to switching off the conscious mind and allowing your trained subconscious to act appropriately. This also promotes a calm, unafraid reaction to the situation, which promotes the full application of technique, uninhibited by the debilitating tenseness of fear.

Fear can be a great enemy, but it can also be your friend. If you do not practice scenario training, the fear of the unknown can have a paralyzing effect. On the other hand, it also provokes the fight or flight response, which gears the body instantly into an optimum state for combat.

Your body and mind interact. If you cower away from an attack in your mind, your body will follow. If you act decisively in your mind, your body will reflect this.

2. Always use methods of distraction—not sometimes but *always*! You are not being attacked by a body, but by a body under the control of a mind. To gain an advantage, disturb his thinking. In ancient Japanese warrior tracts, this would be termed forcing the enemy to have a "stopping mind." Break his concentration and force a moment of uncertainty, at which instant you begin your defensive counter.

The distraction can take many forms: a sudden fierce yell, a sharp unexpected kick to a shin, spitting in the face. All of these and more should form an integral feature of defensive tactics.

3. Control the fighting distance. Never allow a potential enemy into your personal space unless by invitation. In a self-defense situation, your hands should be raised in a protective, non-threatening fashion, which is actually one way to make sure that if an attack occurs, it will be at the target you offer. In other words, trap the assailant into attacking an apparent weakness, whereas in fact you are prepared and ready to immediately take advantage of the attack.

4. Use *metsuke no heiho*. This is an important concept of de-focusing your vision so that your eyes take in all aspects of the enemy, not "stopping" on any particular feature. This non-specific seeing was endorsed by the famous Zen master Takuan Soho (1573–1646) in letters to Yagyu Tajima No Kami Munenori (1571–1646), head of the Yagyu Shinkage-Ryu, dealing with the use of the sword.

This unfocused stare will allow your mind to flow freely and thus act in a disassociated manner without conscious thought intervening. The stare is particularly important if you are in an area where you may run into multiple attackers. One of the features of reaction to extreme stress is the state of hypervigilence, in which the vision becomes "tunneled" and there is a marked loss of peripheral vision. One way to mitigate this is to keep the head moving from side to side, not becoming fixated on any one area for more than a moment.

5. Commit yourself, body and soul, to your defense. Do not be timid and hold back. Never retreat physically or mentally once the combat is inevitable and fighting distance attained (unless it is safe to do so, or as a tactic in order to surprise the enemy).

In the words of Musashi, "Go straight to the heart of your enemy!…It is always best to attack straight ahead.

Your attack must be filled with conviction and purpose. In this way you defeat the enemy regardless of his abilities. This does not mean that straight-in attacks have no circular movements. Research this well!"

6. Never stop until it is over. Even in the least severe situation, if you remain in the area of the attacker and you have only temporarily incapacitated him, it may not be over yet. When executing techniques, do not stop until you are absolutely certain that they have had the desired effect. If a weapon has been involved, at the very least try to ensure that you have control of it.

When the attacker who moments before was trying to deceive you into being off-guard so that he could mug or assault you is finally in your grip, he may promise never to do anything like this again and "gives up." I'm sure you'll believe every word he says!

7. Always move to a position of advantage. In general terms, this means using the color-code awareness procedure so that potential danger can be recognized and avoided altogether. Originally devised by firearms expert Jeff Cooper in the late 1960s, the colors white, yellow, orange and red are used to signify states of mental alertness. (Later, this code has also been applied to levels of danger.) White signifies a relaxed and unprepared state of mind, yellow denotes relaxed but alert, orange communicates awareness of potential danger, and red marks the final stage of combat preparedness. Being in a position of advantage, therefore, does not just apply to a physical position, but also to a mental condition.

In World Wars I and II, British fighter and bomber pilots were warned "Beware of the Hun in the Sun!" (The German fighter pilots had learned to attack the Allied aircraft by diving on them from above and "out of the sun" so that they were almost impossible to see.) Strategically move to the best place from which to defend yourself and make use of local objects as weapons—rocks, trash cans, anything at all.

When the assault commences, remember that outside his bodyline gives you easiest control, whereas the inside position demands faster, more immediate and aggressive action for the defender. Either position is fine, but be sure that you understand the differences.

8. Use the attacker's strength against him, either by unbalancing or deflecting him. This is not just the basic principle of judo, but a common principle in all effective defensive systems. Through judicious use of the pressure points, it is not difficult to invoke the flinch reflex in the attacker's body and force him into an unbalanced position, making it difficult for him to deliver blows with any power. Unbalancing him also places him in the right position for your counter. It is also possible to make the assailant add to his own downfall by, for example, jerking his head violently into the path of your counterattack, thus making your strike even more powerful than it would have been otherwise.

9. Use the vital (vulnerable) areas of the attacker's body to assist techniques. This should go without saying. However, I am amazed at how frequently students forget to target the vital points and end up relying on strength alone, which is foolish in the extreme, especially when one sees how much difference using the points makes. It comes down to serious practice. Too often, dojo training tries to cover too many techniques in one session. It is far better to take just a few techniques and continue to train them for at least 15 minutes or more each. Only after this time will the techniques begin to become a part of muscle memory, and the ability to target the points each and every time becomes part of a natural reaction.

This lack of correct practice is the price paid when karate entered Japan and Funakoshi was persuaded to modify the training to bring it under the influence of Master Jigaro Kano and create a *do* form as Kano had done (Kano had devised a *do* form of ju-jutsu). Most dojos throughout the world now practice and teach this modified, sport form of the original defensive art, to the extent that it is, sadly, almost useless as effective self-defense. Basing training on competition rules can never equal training reflecting the rule-less environs of the street.

10. Never fight at the same speed as the assailant. Usually move much faster to avoid playing catch-up, and sometimes slower to deceive. This is common sense. If an assailant begins an attack, then he already has the advantage. You must learn to react at very high speed in order to negate this advantage. Your defense should be explosive in character.

11. Never give a clue as to your intention. Keep stone-faced. This is something that needs practice. Sometimes your safety may depend upon delivering a pre-emptive strike. You will have only one chance to do this, so it is essential that you give no clue as to your intention beforehand.

12. Show no fear (unless as a tactic). Be prepared to dominate the aggressor psychologically as well as physically.

13. Control your own breathing. In any situation, you can regain control of your physiological responses this way. The fight or flight response to shock can imitate sensations of fear caused by the unknown. In most cases, beginning a slow, deep, rhythmic breathing pattern can help the body to overcome the debilitating effects because it is suddenly not in an unknown situation, but is practicing something for which it has prepared.

14. Do not rely upon any one technique or blow to win the fight. It is unlikely that any single technique will end the confrontation, so be prepared to press your advantage as hard as you can until the assailant is not in a position to continue to attack you.

15. Vary the targets of your strikes. It is frequently much more useful to deliver a hard shin or knee kick to a leg point and then continue with a follow-up strike to the neck, head or arm. This can have a devastating effect and can certainly cause unconsciousness and loss of mobility. Plus there is a great surprise factor if the first thing an aggressor feels of your counter is an unstoppable, unbalancing kick to the inside of his ankle, immediately followed by a knee to his face as he falls forward.

16. When striking, penetrate deeply using the "heavy hand" concept. Following through, rather than stopping the delivery of the blow too soon, ensures maximum power from the strike. Many of the strikes depend on generating a fluid shock effect to the nervous system. By maintaining longer contact and increasing pressure to a vulnerable area of the body, the nerves continue to fire their pain messages over a longer period and with greater urgency, thus strengthening the reaction to the stimulus.

17. If an attacker grabs one arm, use that to unbalance him and pull him into any defensive blow with the other arm, thus increasing the power of the strike. This specifically explains the correct use of the withdrawing hand (*hikite*) in modern karate practice, which currently serves no function whatsoever and places the puncher in an extremely vulnerable position.

18. Use the weapon nearest to the target. In practice, you will frequently find a defender stooping over a fallen attacker in order to use his hands—the feet are invariably closer. Concomitant with this rule is the point that frequently people preparing to punch will first draw back the fist before delivering the blow. This should never happen in defensive situations. Always strike from wherever the hand/fist is currently positioned (hopefully in the hands-up, non-threatening paradigm). This will shorten the time taken to deliver a strike by many tenths of a second, which can be of paramount importance.

To mangle an old English saying: "Thrice armed he whose cause is just: but stronger he whose blow is fust!"

19. Do not hesitate. Prepare a psychological "switch" in your head and be prepared to use it. ("It is not the dog in the fight that matters, rather the fight in the dog!") Any half-hearted response will be almost doomed from the start. Be prepared for the all-too-common denial reaction, where the brain refuses to believe that this incident is occurring and thinks of all sorts of different things (embarrassment, wearing nice clothes) that will stop your correct reaction. Irrational thoughts can cloud the issue, which demands clear thinking and direct action. It *can* happen to you, and *it is* happening to you—deal with it!

20. If you are brought to the ground, get up as quickly as is humanly possible. Avoid fighting on the ground at all costs. You may well be a champion in MMA or ju-jutsu, but it is frequently the case that an assailant has friends who will be eager to play soccer with your head.

21. Always keep your hands moving. When holding your hands up in the non-threatening, compliant position, always keep them moving in a forwards and backwards motion. This will make it impossible for the attacker to notice immediately when your counterstrikes begin. This buys you valuable tenths of a second before the true nature of your movement is recognized.

22. When the opponent is defeated—be careful! The old samurai warrior adage remains true: "When the battle is over, tighten your helmet straps!" When the immediate threat has ended, it is all too easy to allow an enemy the opportunity to attack again when your defenses are down.

I interject a personal reminiscence here that serves to make the point. One night in a nightclub, I was at the foot of some stairs when two struggling figures came rolling down them. They were both worse for drink and grappling away, not doing any harm to each other so I considered it was not my place to interfere, but I deflected their flailing bodies away from a group of ladies that they were about to barge into.

No bouncers arrived and suddenly the situation changed dramatically as one managed to pin the other down and, while strangling him with his own necktie with one hand, somehow removed a shoe and was beating him about the face with it. I had no alternative but to pull him off.

He then swung a punch at me. I deflected it with a circular block, closed on him, trapped his punching arm and lowered him onto his back. As I felt in no danger, there was no necessity to inflict any damage on him so, while pressing his punching arm across his throat, I placed the tip of my index finger on his eye and suggested he think carefully about continuing.

After a moment, he indicated that he had indeed had enough, so I released him. In a flash, as soon as he got to his feet, he swung another punch at my head, so we repeated the entire process, except that on the way down I bounced him gently into the wall.

With my finger once again resting on his eyeball (this, by the way, is an accepted method of bringing down the heart rate and thus his temper—as well as being food for thought), he considered the situation again and decided, no doubt, that if I could do it twice I could probably do it all evening, so after I allowed him up again he wandered off.

The moral of this is simply that if I had "unlaced my helmet straps," so to speak, there is every chance that I would have been caught by surprise. The eventual outcome was that later that evening he came to me and apologized, and thanked me for not hurting him when I obviously could have done so.

Safety in Training

All martial arts training carries a degree of danger. Striking and manipulating the vital points increases the risk of injury, and so it is necessary to develop a consistent and safe approach to all training.

There is another consideration. In normal sports-oriented karate training, the most dangerous targets are banned, but the power of the techniques—even if not aimed specifically at kyusho points—can cause injury. Because of this, much of the training in counterattacking is unnatural in that only light contact is made with the attacker. This leads to the phenomenon of "dojo compliance."

Briefly, this means that in any attack, the assailant maintains good control and never strikes the defender with full power. In Japanese karate, the skill of *sundome* ("stopping very close to the target") is considered a sign of mastery. The effect of this is that the "victim" is never really struck hard, and thus his or her body never reacts in the same way as it would if the blow had actually made hard contact. There is no real pain nor loss of balance, and mental faculties are undisturbed. In exactly the same fashion, the defender never counterattacks by making contact with real force.

When techniques rely on the human body's reaction to force applied to specific points, this can frequently cause difficulties. For example, very often, a good tactic to disable an opponent is to deliver a hard knee strike to the points on the outer thigh. If done in reality, it causes the instantaneous reflex buckling of the leg as the body attempts to move the limb away from the danger and pain. This immediately makes the attacker drop into a lower stance, thus exposing the target (the knockout points on the head) to the follow-up decisive strike. In addition to opening up the target, the head moves towards the blow, thus adding extra force to the impact.

Actually delivering a forceful blow to the initial leg points would clearly be inappropriate in a dojo setting and would certainly cause injury and pain. To mitigate against this, in Kissaki-Kai we use a special thigh pad, which can be moved to cover both the inside and outside of the thigh as required. This allows some degree of force to be delivered and helps to create the correct reaction in the attacker, without which the whole purpose of using the points is missed.

In all of the training, it is important to ensure that the attacker and defender always move their bodies as if they had really been struck and pushed off-balance, just as they would in reality. If this is not done, then no real benefit will accrue from the training, which should always mirror reality as much as is safely possible. In the same way, remember that heads, when struck or punched, invariably move. Many times I see students delivering a punch just short of the attacker's face, but the attacker just stands there, unmoving. This is poor training, and makes it next to impossible for the defender to deliver the next decisive technique because the assailant's head (and therefore his body, too) is not in the correct position. Many kyusho techniques work to create an opening, an exposed target, for a conclusive strike. If the initial blow creates no response, the subsequent technique is negated.

Wearing pads over the arm and leg points enables a more realistic application of force, and creates a limited body reaction that allows for more realistic training. Even so, care should be taken to restrict the degree of force applied as the pads cannot stop the force from being delivered—they only limit it. Safety for one's partner is a paramount concern at all times.

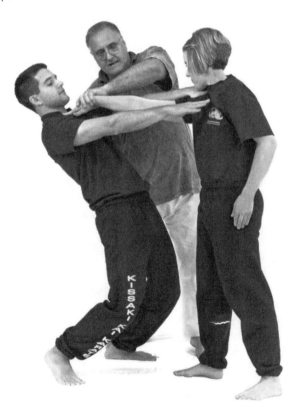

There are certain areas that can be struck with moderate force under strictly controlled conditions, one such being the brachial plexus. I stress, however, that this should only be carried out in the presence of a third observer, and following a sequence of controlled strikes starting from the lightest to the heaviest, which, on a scale of 1 to 10, is never more than level 5 or 6. This type of training I usually reserve for law-enforcement officers and high-ranked martial artists. It should be undertaken only by fit individuals with no health problems. The objective is not to cause unconsciousness, but to evaluate the degree of force generally required in order to temporarily stun an assailant. This is important in the military and law-enforcement environment since, unless one has full confidence in the effectiveness and safety of a technique, it is unlikely that under stress it would ever be used. Therefore, in these circumstances, it is permissible to strike with a little force— never, however, with full power.

Rules of Kyusho Jutsu

- At no time strike your partner hard.
- *Never* cause unconsciousness.
- Mostly use "heavy hands" penetration.
- Practice for speed and smooth application of technique, one flowing into the next.
- Multiple fast strikes serve numerous functions, among which are

  allowing for less than perfect conditions and execution,

  disturbing the balance and mind of the attacker,

  sending multiple pain stimuli to the spine and brain,

  using the reflex mechanism to move the attacker into a position of weakness and vulnerability.

It goes without saying that some targets—the eyes, groin, neck, etc.—should never be struck. It is too dangerous. However, this imposes an even greater responsibility to create a practice scenario in which the attacker reacts appropriately to simulated blows to these areas in order for the training to be realistic. Being a good *uke* ("receiver of the technique") is an art in itself.

Sensible precautions should always be taken in martial training, and it is especially important when the training is as realistic as possible. Add the danger inherent in the use of the vulnerable areas of the body and it should be obvious that all scenarios must be worked through slowly first in order to correctly analyze the potentially dangerous elements. Then, when this has been done, the defenses should be carried out slowly, then with increasing speed (though making sure the techniques can still be carried out safely), until the practice reflects the pace and stress of real life.

Some techniques (strikes, chokes, strangles) are capable of causing unconsciousness. It is *never* a good idea to cause loss of consciousness. Unconsciousness is an unnatural condition and the temptation to test out the effectiveness of techniques should be mitigated by common sense. The long-term effects of causing unconsciousness by means of strikes has only been tested in the sport of boxing, where the state is generally induced by blunt trauma to the head. This has been shown to cause considerable damage over a period, and even bring about Parkinson's disease; the commonly heard description of the "punch-drunk" fighter is often not far from the truth.

However, in studies of hundreds of cases, there has never been any reports of fatalities caused by the bilateral vascular neck restriction type of strangling that cuts off the blood supply to the brain. The reason for this is that the hold is released immediately once the effect is achieved. If the hold were to be maintained for more than the 10-15 seconds usually required, then it is perfectly possible that brain damage could occur.

It is a fundamental concept that you must be responsible for the safety of your training partner.

Revival Techniques

A feature of many performances of knockout techniques by certain "masters" is the application of revival techniques to the unfortunate victim. The flurry of activity, the rush to administer slaps and rubs of dubious merit essentially serves to inculcate the impression that the techniques of the "master" are truly dangerous and effective. In these cases, it is rare that proper unconsciousness occurs. More often than not, the victim is stunned and temporarily disorientated, and would recover perfectly well left on his own. However, the dramatic effect would obviously be somewhat diluted!

The Japanese ju-jutsu systems frequently taught basic revival methods called *kwappo* or *kuatsu*. There are no methods—to my knowledge—that are superior to the commonly taught first-aid techniques of modern Western medicine. For this reason, everyone training in kyusho jutsu should acquire a basic knowledge of CPR by studying with a recognized group.

In most cases, should loss of consciousness occur, the victim should be laid on the ground and, after checking freedom of airways, placed in the recovery position and watched. Medical attention should always be sought following unconsciousness.

The claims made for the efficacy of the ancient methods of revival are as preposterous as those made by some self-styled "masters" for the effects of the techniques themselves. Commenting on the practice of forcing unconscious victims to have their legs forcibly crossed and pushed into an upright seated position, one recent tome, *Kyusho Jitsu*, states: "The seated position also allows the base of the torso or perineum to directly contact the floor as a grounding point for energy transference." The author also states that the initial procedure demands that the victim has his or her legs folded into the "classic lotus position" (Lord help the unconscious victim with stiff, inflexible legs!).

What exactly does this gobbledygook mean? It serves only to drape the master in the cloak of arcane mysticism. There is no "energy" to be transferred, and why the human backside is a more potent transmitter than the whole body prone on the ground is never explained. Such unmitigated, unscientific and wholly unproven nonsense should be ignored. Modern Western first-aid techniques are more than adequate and do not give an opportunity to inflict further harm to a comatose individual who may have a severe neck or spinal injury.

Develop a critical eye. Ask yourself whether such ill-considered advice will serve to protect you in any legal proceedings that may follow any episode which turns bad. My best advice is to attend one of the many courses provided by the Red Cross or some other local outfit. In essence, it will probably include CPR training and suggestions to do very little after checking breathing and airways, with the victim perhaps turned into the recovery position. In any case of loss of consciousness, the only safe course is to obtain proper medical assistance.

How should you train
for optimum results?

Training for real encounters is quite different from regular dojo training. It is always advisable to wear protective equipment, and to be careful to minimize the danger factors by running through scenarios slowly at first so that all parties know precisely what to expect. The actual attacks should mimic reality as much as is safely possible, and should include the swearing and foul language that invariably accompanies certain types of aggressive behavior. The shock effect of abusive language should not be underestimated.

In terms of "how often," the old phrase "Use it or lose it!" is very appropriate. A psychomotor skill is defined as muscular movement resulting from a mental process. The mental component is concerned with decision-making, and the process is an acquired ability to perform defined tasks in response to sensory stimuli. In other words—skill derives from your training. Because it is an acquired or learned skill, it can also be lost or forgotten. If the integrity of the skill is compromised, its effectiveness is devalued.

In 1999, the San Francisco Police Department conducted a series of tests to establish the retention factor in acquired skills. The number of officers taking part in the test was 121. The test itself had three parts: control hold, pat-down search, and handcuff technique.

The level of complexity involved in the performance of the techniques had a significant effect upon the level of retention. For example, control hold criteria include mechanical function, balance, and the controlling force and the appropriateness of the procedure.

Those officers who had received training in control holds within the previous 12 months scored 70 percent at an acceptable level of performance, leaving 30 percent below the acceptable level. Those officers who hadn't had training for 24 months scored 63 percent at an acceptable level, with 37 percent below the acceptable level.

Only 31 percent of officers who hadn't had training for more than 24 months scored at an acceptable level.

Both the search and handcuffing criteria were more complex, including approach and awareness, foot movement, balance, controlling force, mechanics, verbal instruction, and appropriateness. As can be seen in the table and confirmed by other studies, if a technique is relatively simple, after a 12-month period the retention rate is about 70 percent. However, if the procedure is more complex (as the training in verbal dissuasion from aggression would demand), then the retention rate falls to a lower unacceptable level, assuming there is no retraining factor.

Retention of Acquired Skills

Technique	Control Hold	Handcuffing	Search
12 Months	70%	65%	47%
12–24 Months	63%	57%	44%
24+ Months	31%	34%	36%

This study was aimed at police officers who were carrying out these techniques frequently in the course of their regular duties. In light of this, it is significant that just repeating an action without critically assessing the performance and re-instituting corrections does not maintain optimum skill levels. Doing something incorrectly over and over again only makes it more likely that you will do it wrong again next time.

Therefore, for officers and civilians who desire to enhance their defensive techniques using the vital points, it is even more important that the techniques be returned to and practiced very frequently. From my own observations of hundreds of students over the years, I am continually dismayed by the numbers of them who can point to a vulnerable area in practice, but who do not make correct use of it under pressure and stress.

The answer is to practice over and over again just a few of the more important techniques until the reaction to attack is spontaneous and correct. Then go back and spend time on them every few weeks to make sure the response is sharp and accurate.

PART 2:
COMBAT
APPLICATIONS

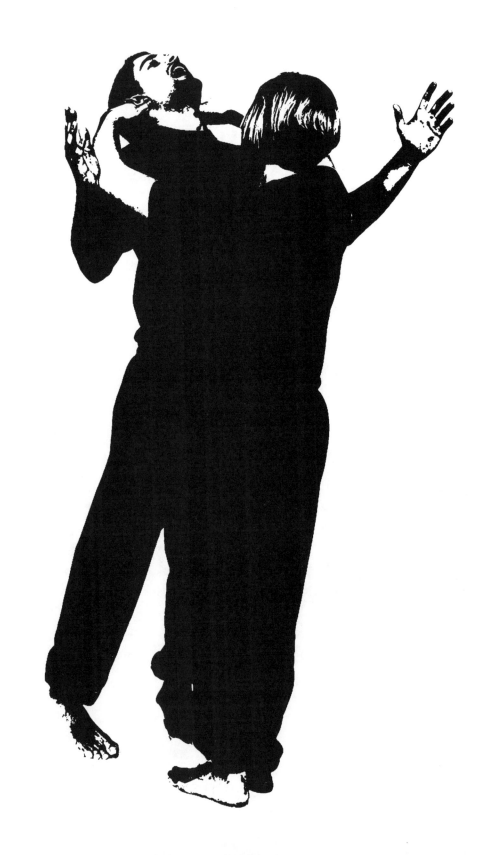

COMBAT
APPLICATIONS

This section covers single and combination techniques against a variety of commonly occurring assaults. The physical structure of human beings dictates the small number of anatomical weapons that can be used in any attack or assault situation. The nature of the assault, robbery, rape, violence and participants (male versus male, male versus female) will further dictate the type of attack. A secondary consideration will be whether or not a weapon is involved and, if so, what type (e.g., firearm, edged weapon, blunt instrument).

Although the details of any specific attack will vary, in general assailants consistently employ similar weapons and methods of attack throughout the world. This being so, it is possible to categorize them into attacks with commonly occurring features and thus devise defensive techniques against them, following the Rule of Combat: "Learn to defend against the most likely and common form of attack first."

Low-level violence
Wrist and arm grabs
Wrist and arm grabs can be merely minor irritations, but they can also escalate to a much more serious level of attack. The potential severity of the assault must be judged and the defense selected accordingly. (It is possible to select a defense at this level of attack because the fear factor and physiological response will not take the body into the state of hypervigilance, which renders the brain unable to make selective decisions.) This is a common feature in domestic violence disputes and is also a standard opening tactic in attempted abductions. The Rules of Combat—as always—apply. Notice that although only wrist grabs are shown, these techniques work just as well for arm grabs.

Slaps

The slap is often considered to be of very minor importance in the hierarchy of striking techniques and it can often be seen used ineffectually when two untrained women have a drunken spat. However, if used effectively, it can be a major weapon very capable of causing a knockout. In fact, one of my colleagues has, in the real world, used it to render assailants unconscious, striking hard to the ear drum or the points on the side of the face and head. When an assailant has chosen this technique, it should not therefore be treated any more lightly than if it were a punch.

More-violent situations
Grabbing and molestation

As these are potentially more dangerous situations, you must be prepared to act decisively and quickly with no hesitation and deliver blows with full force. If you fail to do this, your retaliation may serve to escalate the level of violence instead of controlling it. In most of these instances, it will be necessary to incapacitate the attacker before leaving the scene so that he is unable to continue the attack.

Sudden attacks

If an assault is truly unexpected, the shock of an attacker suddenly moving to grab or strike will invoke a reflexive response in the victim. Characteristically this will involve a ducking motion while bringing the hands up in a defensive position. This unconscious reaction can be very effective in allowing the victim to survive the first chaotic and surprising moment of the assault. It is a good idea to build a defensive paradigm based on the body's natural reactions because these always take place, no matter what. The body's reflexive response can also be put to good use in defensive techniques (see jab to throat, pages 48 and 71). The attacker's automatic reflexive reaction to these techniques will force him to release his grip immediately and turn his body away from the source of the attack.

Life-threatening situations
Abduction

In an attempted abduction scenario, you want to compromise your attacker's ability to move as much as possible so that once you have attained your initial escape, the attacker cannot pursue or attack you again.

Strangling or choking

Choking or strangulation is one of the most common violent attacks leading to the death of the victim. Obviously, this type of attack has to be dealt with immediately. Any delay will leave the body too weak to effect a defense.

On the ground

In the world of martial arts, as in the general world, there are trends, fads and fashions. Following the phenomenon that was Bruce Lee, karate and kung fu became popular. Later came Gracie Brothers ju-jutsu and, with the spread of Mixed Martial Arts, the current trend is towards fighting on the ground.

It is undeniable that MMA fighters are strong, skillful and extremely good at what they do. Do not, however, confuse this brutal sport with reality. It is not! If you carefully watch any of the televised bouts of even the most extreme groundfighting, you will see that there are still rules in operation. Many of the hold-downs, which allow the fighter in the mount position to deliver successive elbow strikes and punches, would be impossible if the defender were allowed to attack the eyes with finger strikes, bite the ears and neck, and pinch the vulnerable arm points. It is also worth noting that direct attacks to the back of the neck are forbidden, as is the twisting and breaking of fingers and headbutts to the face.

Were both combatants allowed to make use of these forbidden (ipso facto, extremely effective) techniques, then the fights would look completely different. Of course, this could never happen as the dangers to the participants are obvious. This should make anyone interested in real self-defense stop and think before devoting their time to MMA practice.

In the streets there are no rules, and frequently there are multiple opponents. It is therefore never a good idea to go to the ground with an attacker. You may indeed be a champion wrestler or ju-jutsuka and you may well be holding your own or even beating your assailant, but you never know how many friends he has until their boots use your head as a football. However, if the attack is an attempted rape or sexual assault, you will already be where the attacker wants you to be. If you are a law-enforcement official, it is likely that you have strapped to your body a variety of bulky objects that will impede your ability to roll and twist effectively on the ground; in all circumstances, your strategy is to regain your footing as quickly as possible. The tactics by which you do so will depend to a great extent on the type of attack in progress.

In all circumstances where the defender has to gain a standing position, it is important that all practice is done without using the hands to facilitate this as they may be needed to perform a defensive or attacking function at the same time. Using the hands to aid in regaining a standing position therefore allows opportunity for the aggressor to attack again.

Offensive Techniques
Chokes and strangles

The most common method of murder or causing death with bare hands is by manual strangulation, as illustrated in the previous scenarios. Loss of consciousness and death is generally caused by a crushing pressure on the front of the throat, deforming the trachea and usually breaking the hyoid bone, thus obstructing the airways.

There are indeed chokes that, when used as defensive techniques, affect the airways and cause death in the same manner. These are in the main only to be used in the most desperate of situations and are, frankly, unnecessary since techniques that affect the flow of blood to the brain can bring about the same effects without any of the same dangers.

Scenario: The assailant seizes your right wrist with either hand in an attempt to intimidate or drag you.

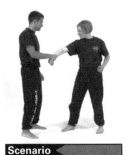

Scenario

Strategy: Obtain release from the grip and escape from the area.

Tactics:

1 Perform a distraction technique (by either shouting, screaming, spitting, kicking or slapping).

2 Move at a 45-degree angle to the attacker and pull to unbalance him. Strike vital point Lu.7 on the attacker's wrist using a hammerfist or the outside edge of your lower forearm, and pull strongly to effect the release.

Leave the scene.

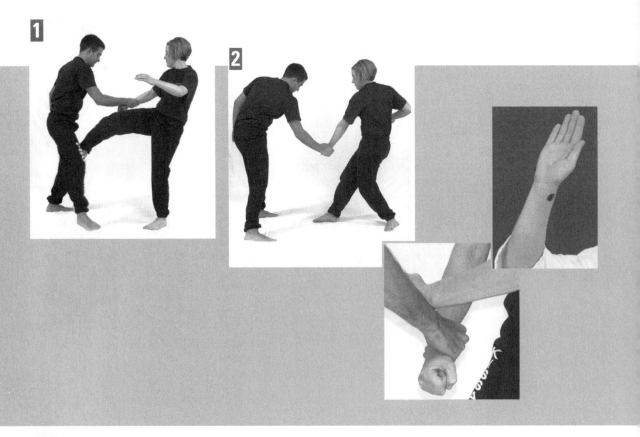

Wrist and arm grabs

Scenario: *The assailant seizes either wrist and pulls to the side.*

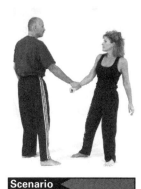

Strategy: Obtain release from the grip, disable the attacker and escape from the area.

Tactics:

1 Go with the pull and perform a distraction technique (by either striking, shouting or screaming).

2 Drive either knee into the Gb.32 points on the attacker's outer thigh.

3 Follow up immediately with a palm heel strike to the attacker's ear.

Leave the scene.

Scenario

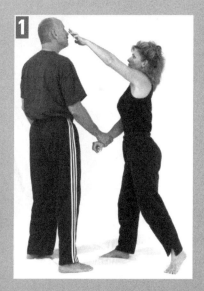

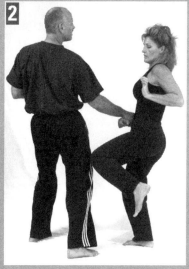

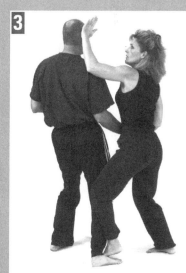

While the overall strategy is still to escape from the assailant, in this instance the attacker is temporarily incapacitated by a Kyusho strike to the arm (Tw.12), which can bring him to his knees if executed correctly. It is crucial to strike with the concept of "heavy hands," as described in the Rules of Combat section; if this is not done, the technique is unlikely to put the attacker down.

Scenario: *The assailant seizes your left wrist with his left hand in an attempt to intimidate, strike or drag you.*

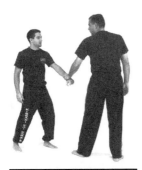

Scenario

Strategy: Obtain release from the grip, disable the attacker and escape from the area.

Tactics:

1 Perform a distraction technique (by either shouting, screaming, spitting, kicking or slapping).

2 Unbalance the attacker by moving to a position of advantage to the outside of the attacker's centerline, away from his other hand; at the same time, twist the attacker's arm clockwise to expose the Tw.12 point.

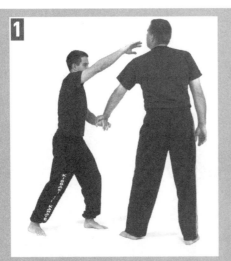

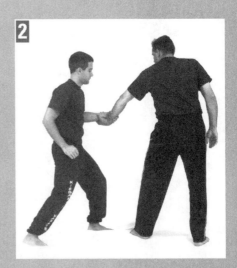

3 Strike the vital point on the back of the attacker's arm, at mid-triceps level, with a hammerfist or the outside edge of your lower forearm.

4 Pull your other hand in the direction opposite to the counterstrike to effect the release; driving your forearm right through the point will knock the assailant to the ground, leaving his arm in position to apply a control hold if required.

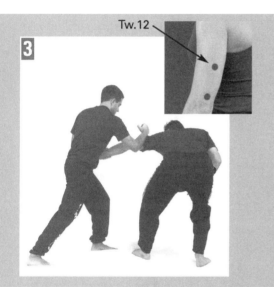

Tw.12

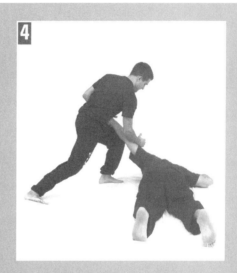

Variation: In the event that the first strike to the attacker's Tw.12 point is not powerful enough to knock him to the ground immediately, slide your right leg in front of the attacker's left leg and, continuing to push down firmly on his arm, sweep away his nearest leg with the back of your right leg to drive him to the ground.

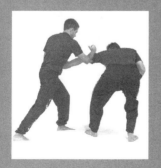
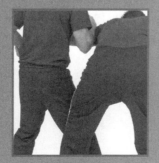
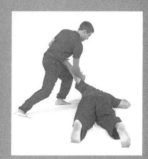

Scenario: *The assailant seizes you by both shoulders and begins shaking you.*

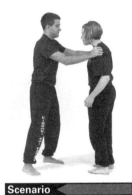

Scenario

Strategy: Obtain release from the grip, disable the attacker and escape from the area.

Tactics:

1 Perform a distraction technique (by either shouting, screaming, spitting or kicking).

2 Bring one arm up between the attacker's arms and jab your extended fingers into the eyes or throat to obtain release. This will unbalance the assailant and allow you to leave the scene or utilize a follow-up technique if necessary.

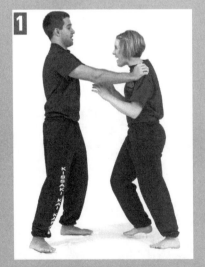

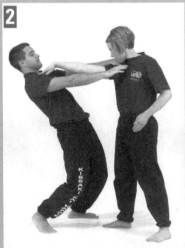

Scenario: The attacker uses both hands to seize you by one wrist and begins pulling.

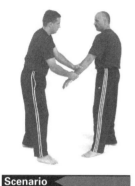

Strategy: Obtain release from the grip, disable the attacker and escape from the area.

Tactics:

1 Perform a distraction technique (by either shouting, screaming, spitting or kicking). Place your free hand under the palm of your captured hand.

2-3 Using your body, twist both hands out to the side and upward.

This will turn the attacker's arms so that his outside arm's elbow rotates upward.

Continued on page 50.

Scenario

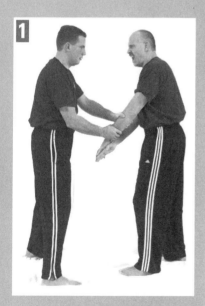

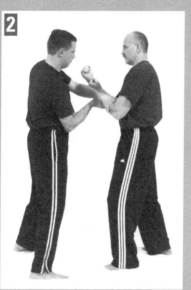

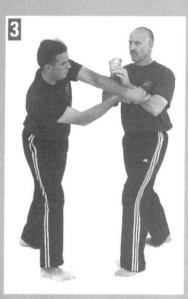

4 Use your captured hand to seize his wrist and form a base as your free hand strikes hard into the Tw.12 point in the middle of his triceps muscle. This will force his legs to buckle and his grip to loosen.

5 Now drive your knee hard into the Gb.31 or Gb.32 point on his thigh to cause him to drop even further forward.

6 At this stage deliver a hard palm heel strike to his ear or Gb.3 or Gb.4 points on the temple to stun him.

Leave the scene.

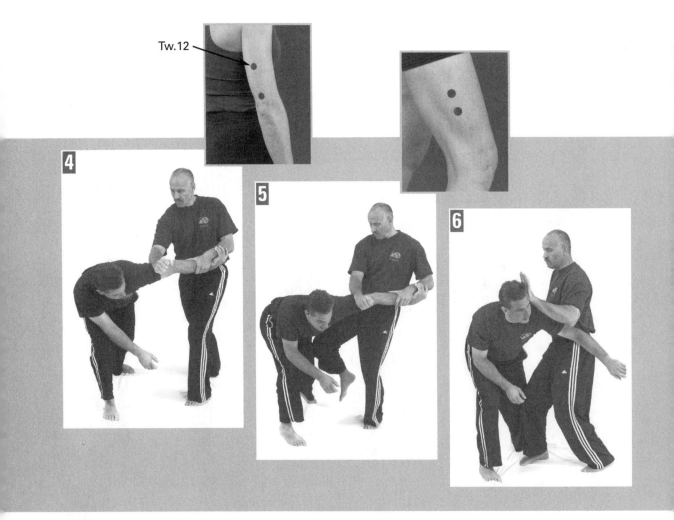

Tw.12

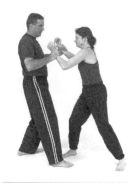

Scenario

Strategy: Obtain release from the grip, disable the attacker and escape from the area.

Tactics:

1 Perform a distraction technique (by either shouting, screaming, spitting or kicking).

2-3 Simultaneously jerk both of your hands wide apart. This will pull the attacker's face close to yours. Lower your chin and drive the top of your head hard anywhere into the attacker's face.

4 As the attacker releases you and reels back from the force of the blow, deliver a hard roundhouse kick with your shin to the Gb.31 point on either of his thighs to disable his leg and affect his mobility.

Leave the scene.

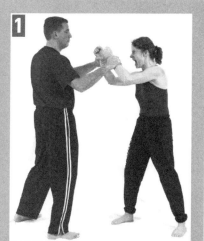

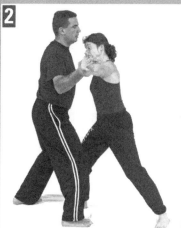

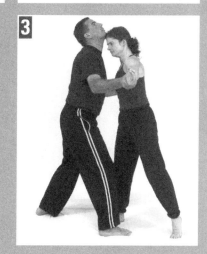

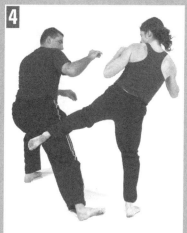

Scenario: The attacker is raising his hand to slap you.

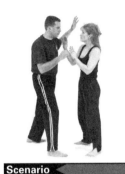

Scenario

Strategy: Prevent the blow to the face from landing,

Tactics:

1. Use the frisbee block: As the attacker begins to swing the slap, move forward and jam the outside of your extended forearm past the attacker's head so that you connect with the vital points on his arm.

This will immediately disable the arm.

2. With the other hand, immediately deliver a palm heel strike under the chin or under the nose. In a more violent situation, strike the attacker's eyes or throat.

Leave the scene.

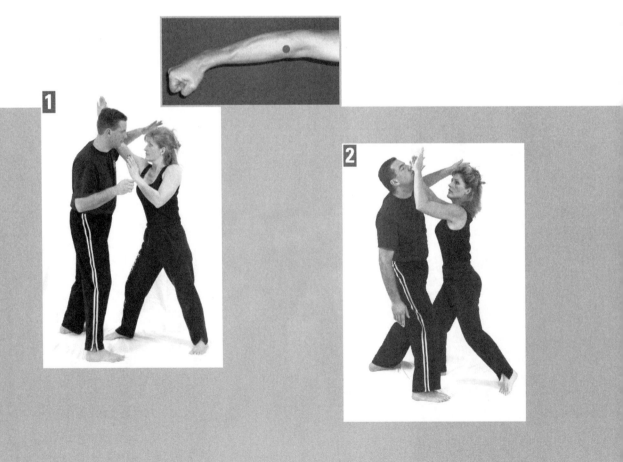

Grabbing and molestation

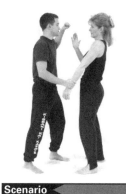

Scenario

This defense allows you to utilize the opponent's force against him, because if you do not hesitate between the block and the slap, you can channel the force of the attacker's blow right back into the attacker's own vital points. This is really a nice point of justice in that the harder the attacker tries to assault you, the more damage he does to himself. Either point strike will create a massive disturbance to the brain and overload the nervous system, especially in conjunction with the hard strike to the arm points which it follows. It is also possible to rupture the ear drum with this technique, so take care in training.

Note that if your awareness levels are operating correctly, this situation should never arise, unless you use it as a tactic to induce the attacker to put himself in a position of your choice. At the very most, this complete defense should be executed within two to three seconds.

Scenario: *The attacker seizes you by the wrist with one hand and attempts to strike your head with the other.*

Strategy: Prevent the blow to the face from landing, obtain release from the grip and temporarily disable the assailant.

Tactics:

1 Use the frisbee block: As the attacker begins to swing the punch, move forward and jam the outside of your extended forearm past the attacker's head so that you connect with the vital points on his arm. This will immediately disable the arm.

2 Without pausing, slap the palm heel of your blocking arm into the Gb.20 point on the back of the attacker's neck or onto the ear, whichever target is presented.

3 If necessary, with the same arm, strike the attacker's gripping arm at the Lu.5 point to effect a release.

Leave the scene.

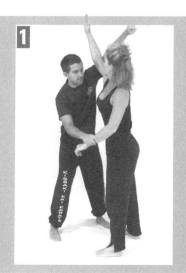

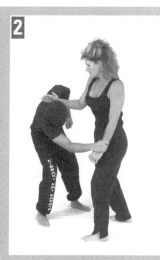

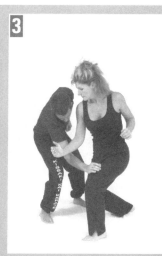

It is perfectly possible to use the same technique as in the previous defense with just a few minor adjustments.

Scenario: *The attacker seizes you by the lapel or shirt front with his left hand and attempts to strike your head with his right.*

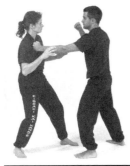

Scenario

Strategy: Prevent the blow to the face from landing and control the hand gripping the lapel; obtain release from the grip and temporarily disable the assailant.

Tactics:

1 Perform the frisbee block with your left arm: As the attacker begins to swing the punch, move forward and jam the outside of your extended forearm past the attacker's head so that you connect with the vital points on his arm. Simultaneously with your right hand, clasp the attacker's gripping hand tightly to his chest.

This effectively removes one weapon from the attacker's arsenal.

2 As the block impacts the assailant's arm, immediately smack the top of your forehead directly into the attacker's face.

3 As the attacker reels backwards from the force of the blow, follow with a hard palm heel strike with your left arm to the St.5 point on the side of the attacker's jaw. This will either stun him or cause him to lose consciousness.

Leave the scene.

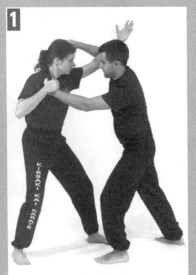

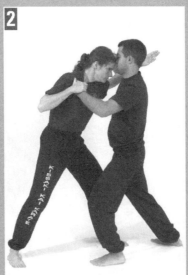

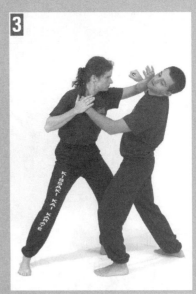

One of the characteristic reactions to vital point strikes to the Lu.5 area is that the head reflexively jerks forward and is therefore presented as a target.

Scenario: The attacker grabs your torso in a bearhug from the front, reaching under both arms in an attempt to intimidate or abduct you.

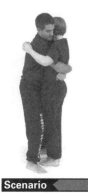

Strategy: Prevent the opponent from crushing your ribs and affecting your breathing, and obtain release.

Tactics:

1 Tighten your stomach muscles, slide both thumbs under the attacker's ear lobes (Tw.17), and jab sharply inward and upward.

As the attacker releases the grip, leave the scene or apply a follow-up technique.

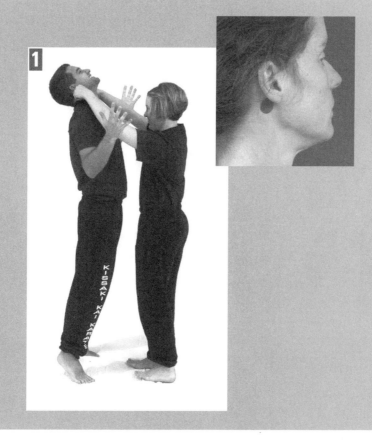

In any situation where both of your arms are trapped either from the front, side or rear, your primary objective is to retain the ability to breathe. You do this by creating a gap between the encircling arms and your own torso by placing your palms on you thighs and straightening your arms by pushing them down towards your knees. Even if you can only create a small gap, that will be enough. The aim is always to force the attacker to relinquish his hold. He will do this as he tires and sees that his grip is not having the desired effect.

Scenario: The attacker grabs your torso in a bearhug from the front, reaching over both arms in an attempt to intimidate or abduct you.

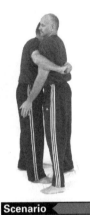

Strategy: Prevent the opponent from crushing your ribs and affecting your breathing, and obtain release.

Tactics:

1-2 Immediately drive both of your arms downward until your arms are on your knees. This creates a gap, which will enable you to continue to breathe. You can facilitate this by first using your hands to slide further downward and pinch the assailant's inner thighs or even directly attack his testicles.

3 As you do this, continually attempt to strike his face with the top of your forehead, as well as stamp on his foot and rake the sole of your foot down his shin to create a response.

Scenario

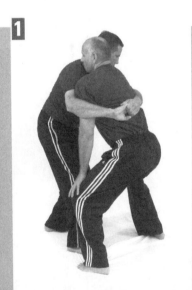

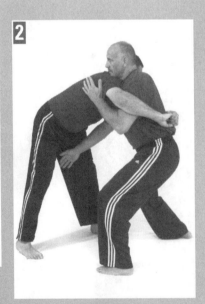

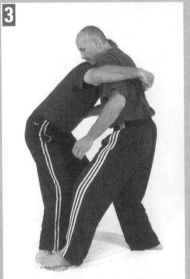

4 Once the grip is released, incapacitate the attacker by twisting slightly to a 45-degree angle (keeping your hands up to protect your face) and driving your heel into the Sp.10 point on the inside of the attacker's thigh. This will invoke a reflex reaction, which will force his body away from you and drop his head downward.

5 Drive the same knee up into his face to stun him.

Leave the scene.

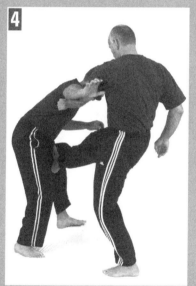

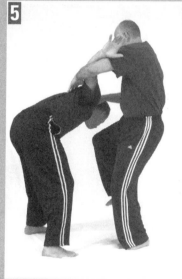

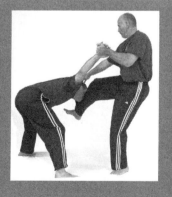

Variation: If your initial thigh kick has moved him slightly further away, deliver a shin kick to his face instead of the knee strike.

Any attack involving seizing and pulling the hair can cause a great deal of pain and confusion in the victim. The head can also be jerked around, stunning the victim.

Scenario: *The attacker grabs your hair from the rear. (This is particularly applicable to women.)*

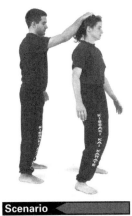

Strategy: Obtain release, disable the attacker and leave the scene.

Tactics:

1 Clamp the attacker's pulling hand firmly to your head with both hands to alleviate the pain.

2 Duck down and turn underneath the attacker's hand so that you are now facing the attacker.

3 Reach up and savagely pinch the flesh on the inside and underside of the attacker's upper arm, which will invoke a flinch-reflex withdrawal reaction and cause the assailant to let go.

Leave the scene.

Scenario ◀

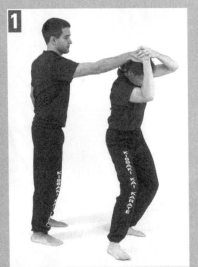

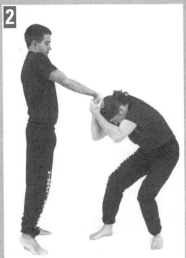

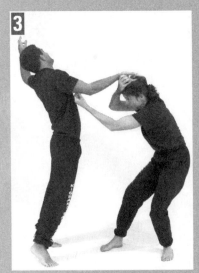

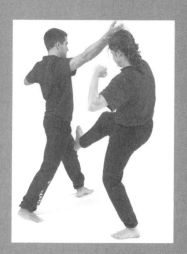

Variation: If the situation feels more serious, after Step 3, immediately deliver a hard heel kick to the Sp.10 or 11 points on the assailant's inner thigh. Follow this with a shin strike to either of the Gb. points on the outside thigh of the other leg. A hard strike here will force the attacker to release his grip as his knee buckles from the blow.

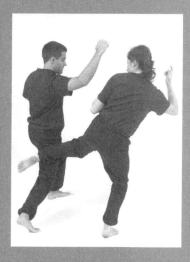

Scenario: *The attacker grabs your hair from the front, but is deemed to be more serious than the prior scenario (Technique 5).*

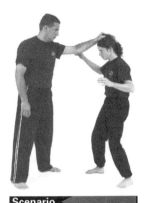

Scenario

Strategy: Obtain release, disable the attacker and leave the scene.

Tactics:

1 Clamp one hand onto the hand gripping your hair and bend forward a little to apply pressure to the assailant's wrist. With your other hand, apply downward pressure to the Lu.5 point to bend the attacker's arm and bring him in range for the following technique.

2 Immediately deliver a hard heel kick to the Sp.10 or 11 points on the assailant's inner thigh.

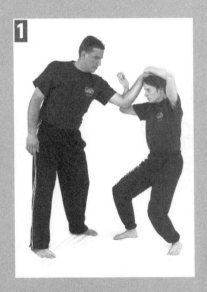

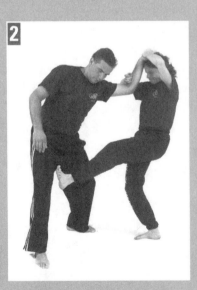

3 Follow this with a shin strike to either of the Gb. points on the outside thigh of the other leg. A hard strike here will force the attacker to release his grip as his knee buckles from the blow.

4 As the attacker's body drops downward and forward, immediately follow up with a roundhouse strike to the Gb.20 point on the back of his head using your nearest elbow. This will stun him or cause unconsciousness.

Leave the scene.

Remember the principle that you really do not need ten different defenses against ten different attacks. It is always better to have one defense that will deal with ten different attacks. In the event of hair being pulled, the first and most common defense feature will be to clamp the pulling hand to the head before applying follow-up defensive maneuvers.

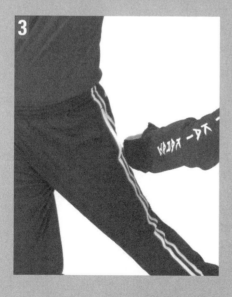

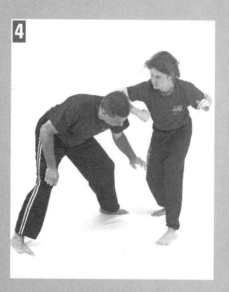

Scenario: *The attacker grabs your lapels or shirt front with both hands and prepares for a headbutt.*

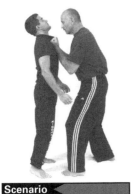

Strategy: Prevent head butt from landing, enable release, temporarily disable the attacker and leave the scene.

Tactics:

1 Perform a distraction technique (by either shouting, screaming or spitting). Simultaneously lower your chin to your chest to offer only the hard target of your forehead or the top of your head to the attacker.

2–3 As he flexes his arms to draw you in close, jab the first two fingers of both hands directly into his eyes. The withdrawal reflex response will force him to pull his head away sharply and release his grip.

Leave the scene.

Scenario

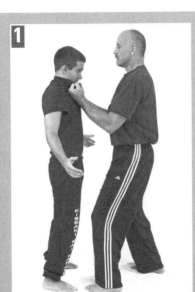

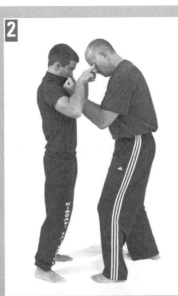

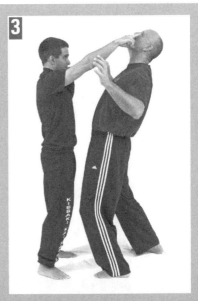

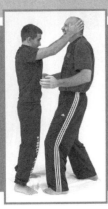

Variation: Drive both thumbs into the attacker's eyes or slap both cupped palms hard onto both the attacker's ears.

Scenario: *The attacker grabs your shoulder and spins you around into his punch.*

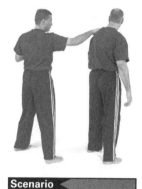

Strategy: Avoid the blow, temporarily disable the attacker and leave the scene.

Tactics:

1-2 As you turn, a reflexive flinch reaction has caused you to raise your hand in front of your face; use this reflex to trigger the fris- bee block. Slam a palm heel strike into the St.5 point at the side of the attacker's jaw for a stun or knockout. This has to be done very quickly, before the attacker's punch has a chance to land.

Scenario

Continued on page 64.

Ignore the arm that grips and pulls the shoulder. A hand that is performing such a function is no immediate danger. It will simply be a waste of time and of one of your weapons to attempt to detach its grip.

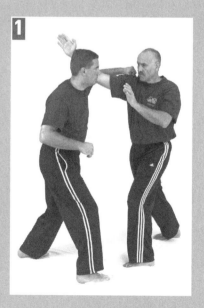

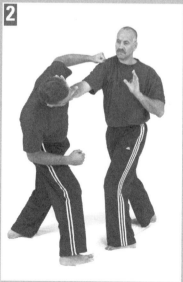

3-4 Immediately seize the St.9 points on either side of the assailant's trachea, pushing sharply upward so that the withdrawal reflex forces the assailant up onto tiptoe.

5 If the pain is not sufficient to halt the attack, quickly release the hold and deliver a strike (palm heel or fist) to the attacker's groin.

6 As the attacker drops downward, drive an elbow strike upward into his jaw for a knockout.

Leave the scene.

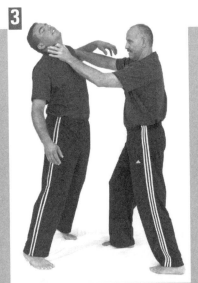

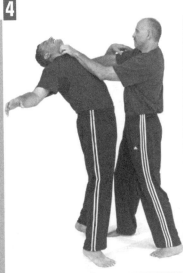

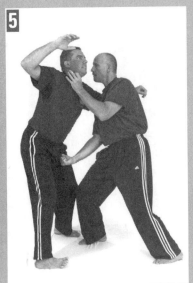

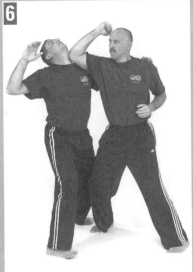

Scenario: *The assailant bearhugs you from behind, reaching under your arms in an attempt to force you to the ground.*

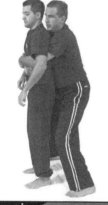

Scenario

Strategy: Obtain release from the grip, temporarily disable the attacker and leave the scene.

Tactics:

1 Immediately tighten your stomach muscles to ensure that you can continue to breathe against the squeezing of the assailant's arms. Now repeatedly drive your head backwards in an attempt to strike the opponent's face—distracting the attacker's concentration on the grip will make it easier to break the grip.

2 At the same time, continuously try to heel-kick the attacker's shins (ideally striking in the area of Sp.6, just above the ankle and to the inside of the leg), drag your heel up and down his shin, and stamp on his foot to distract him.

3 When possible, take hold of his uppermost wrist. If you can grasp one of his little fingers and bend it back, this will also help to break the hold.

Continued on page 66.

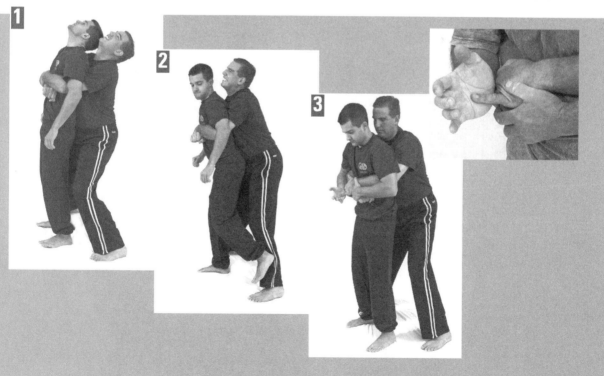

4 As the grip is released, twist the attacker's arm sharply so that the elbow is turned upward as you move to the outside of his centerline.

5 Slam your forearm hard down through the Tw.12 point to buckle his knees. Repeat the strike again to force him to the ground.

Leave the scene.

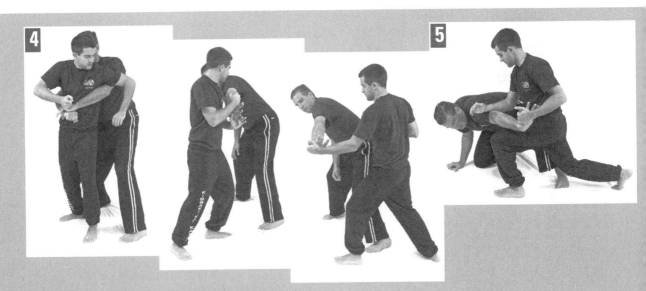

Should the assailant lift you from the ground and attempt to carry you away, there is little you can do in this position. In order to make him put you back on the ground, you must apply all the techniques above as hard and as quickly as you can while continuing to shout, struggle and wriggle. Eventually the attacker will have to put you down, at which point, you can continue the technique as described above.

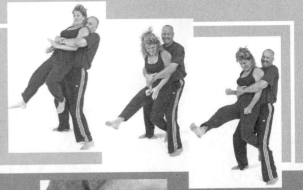

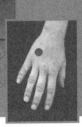

Variation: In a less dangerous situation, you can also distract the opponent by rubbing your thumb joint or knuckle hard into the Tw.3 point on the back of his hand.

Scenario: *The assailant applies a headlock from the side.*

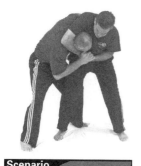

Strategy: Obtain release from the lock, temporarily disable the attacker and leave the scene.

Tactics:

1-2 Using your arm nearest to the attacker's body, circle it up and around him from behind in an attempt to jab your fingers into his eye. This will gain his attention and he will react by pulling his head backwards, away from your fingers. While doing this, slide your other arm either in front or behind the leg nearest to you (whichever is easiest) and start to pinch as hard as you can on the spleen meridian on the inside of his thigh. This double attack will distract his attention from his grip.

Continued on page 68.

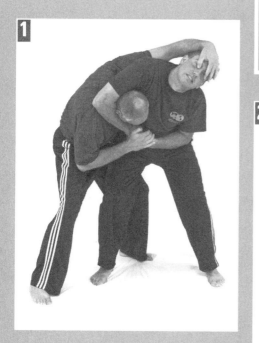

In the struggle, do not waste time by trying to grip the attacker's wrists and levering them open. While his hands are grabbing you, they are not doing anything else, so you have time to use your free weapons to good effect.

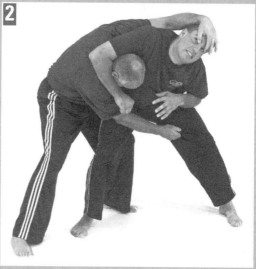

3-4 If the attacker has long-enough hair, stop jabbing his eye and grip his hair on the side of his head furthest away from you—twist and pull back sharply. This will force his head to turn away from you. At this stage, force your body upright while continuing to pull him backwards to the ground by his hair at which point you can apply a control hold if necessary.

Leave the scene.

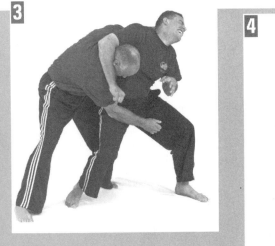

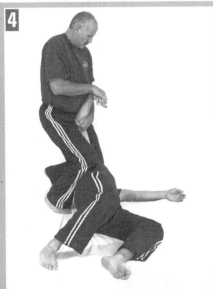

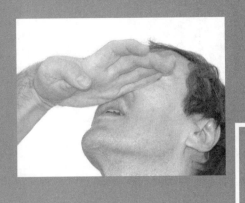

Variation: If the attacker is bald or has very short hair, slide the pinky-edge of your hand underneath his nose and press hard into the pressure point Gv.26 and force his head backward and downward until he falls to the ground.

Scenario: *The assailant seizes you by one wrist and attempts to pull you into a vehicle.*

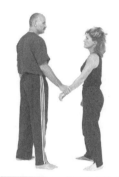

Scenario

Strategy: Use a distraction technique, temporarily disable the attacker and leave the scene.

Tactics:

1 Simultaneously make a distraction technique by snapping one hand hard under the attacker's nose (Gv.26). As the assailant reflexively draws back from the distraction technique, his gripping arm will straighten, revealing the Lu.5 point, which is the target of the next defensive strike.

2-3 Drive your forearm down hard through the Lu.5 point. This will immediately snap the attacker's head forward into the upward forearm strike to the St.5 point on the side of his jaw for a stun or full knockout, depending upon the force of the blow. The technique is executed with speed; by introducing the extra impact gained by adding body weight as you slide away and then back, it becomes very powerful indeed and can easily cause unconsciousness.

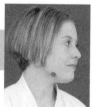

Note: The primary target is the St.5 point on the side of the jaw, but equally effective results can be achieved by striking any of the points at the side of the neck.

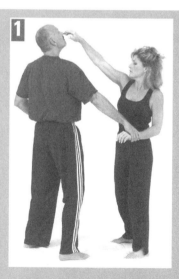

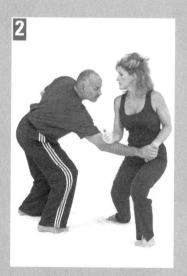

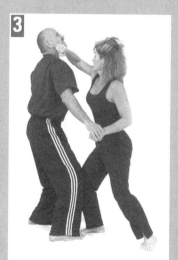

Scenario: The assailant seizes you by one or both arms and attempts to pull you into a vehicle or a dangerous place.

Strategy: Obtain release from the grip, disable the attacker and leave the scene.

Tactics:

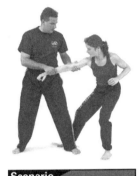

Scenario

1 Pull yourself in towards the attacker and drive your knee hard into the Gb.31 outside-thigh point of the attacker's nearest leg. The effect of the thigh strike will cause the attacker's knees to buckle and drop his head forward.

2-3 Immediately strike hard to his ear or the side of his face or jaw with a palm heel strike. This will stun the aggressor and allow you to twist your own gripped arm so that the assailant's arm is turned elbow upward.

4 Drive your forearm hard down through the Tw.12 point on the back of the attacker's triceps muscle, which will drive him to his knees.

Leave the scene.

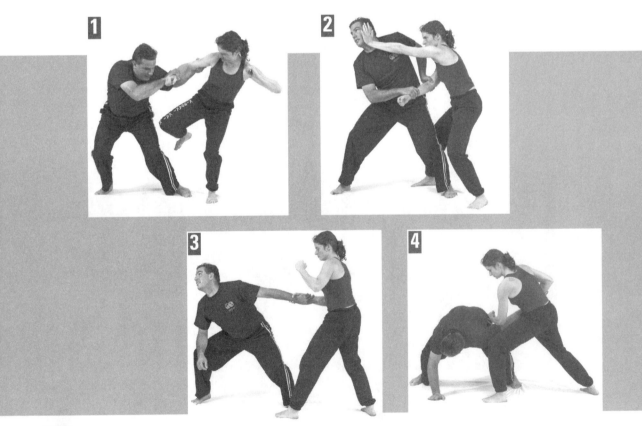

Scenario: *The assailant bearhugs you from behind, reaching over your arms.*

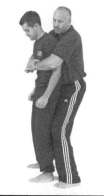

Scenario

Strategy: Obtain release from the grip, temporarily disable the attacker and leave the scene.

Tactics:

1 To ensure that you can continue to breathe, bend your body forward and slide the palms of both hands over both of your knees. Now straighten your arms as strongly as you can. This will force a small gap between the attacker's encircling arms and your torso, thus allowing you to continue to breathe. This position also makes it difficult for the attacker to pick you up.

2-3 As soon as you can, jerk and twist your body while attempting to stamp on the attacker's shin or foot. At the same time, keep driving your head backwards to strike the attacker's face.

Continued on page 72.

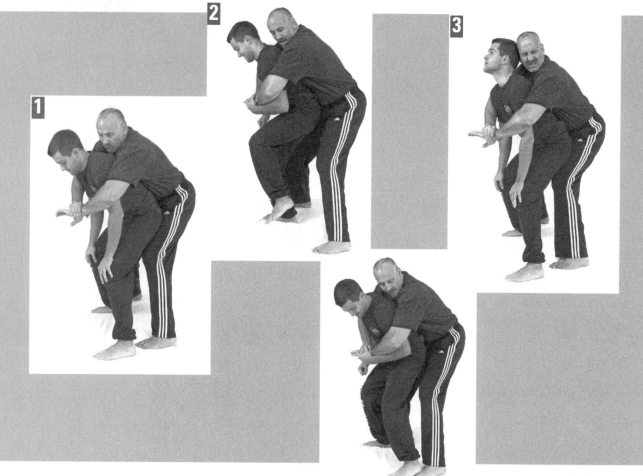

4 As the grip loosens, grab the uppermost wrist and pull it forward as you drive the elbow of your other arm hard into the assailant's torso.

5 If you have done this with your left elbow and are gripping his wrist with your right hand, duck underneath his extended arm and turn clockwise. This will force the attacker to bend forward and keep his arm extended with the elbow upward.

6 Immediately strike down hard with your left forearm through the Tw.12 point on his triceps. This will force him further forward.

7 Drive a kick with your left shin anywhere into his face to stun and incapacitate him.

Leave the scene.

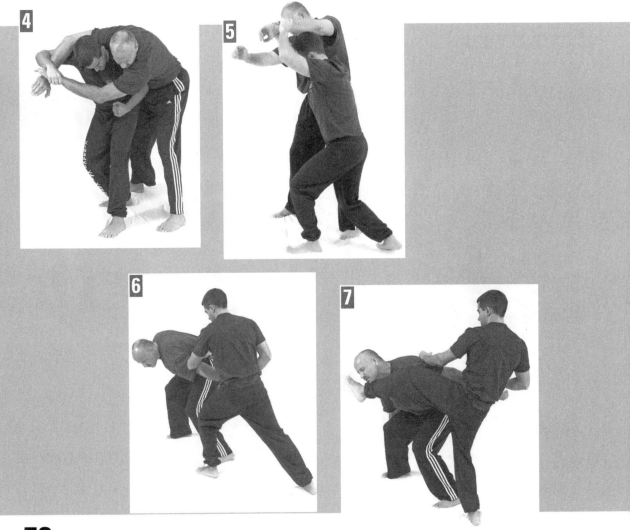

Strangling or choking

Scenario: The attacker seizes you by the throat from the front.

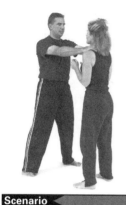

Scenario

Strategy: Obtain release, temporarily disable the attacker and leave the scene.

Tactics:

1 With your fingertips pressed together, bring one hand up between the attacker's arms and drive firmly into the Cv.22 point above the sternal notch on the assailant's throat. At the same time, push yourself away and turn your head sharply as if looking behind. This sharp pressure into the Cv.22 point will invoke a reflex gag response, which will force the assailant to pull backwards and release his grip.

Leave the scene.

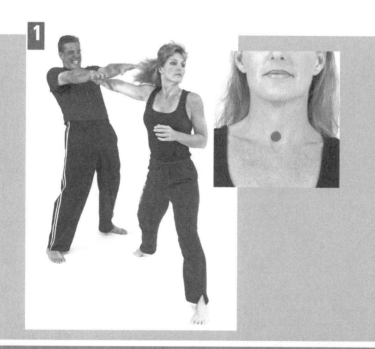

Variation: If the attack is deemed to be more serious, drive a finger deep into one or both of the assailant's eyes. The reaction will be an instant release of his grip and a reflexive turning away of his head and body.

Scenario: *The attacker seizes you by the throat from the front.*

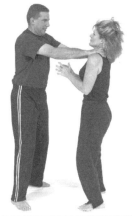

Scenario

Strategy: Obtain release and leave the scene.

Tactics:

1-2 With the forefinger and thumb of both hands, pinch in a sharp upward direction the underside of the attacker's upper arms. The acute pain in this vulnerable area will invoke a reflexive withdrawal response, forcing the attacker to release his grip and jerk his hands away.

Leave the scene.

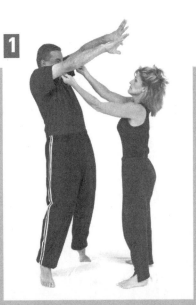
1

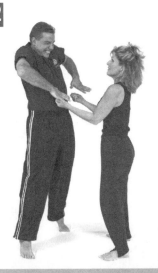
2

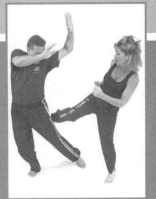

Note that in techniques 1 and 2, the initial defensive techniques are to prevent strangulation. In many instances the assailant's reaction will give the defender time to run. If the situation is more serious, follow-up techniques in the form of kicks or strikes to other vital points must be added. For example, as the assailant involuntarily pulls away from the defender, he will generally expose the Gb.31/Gb.32 points on the thigh, which can be struck hard with the knee or shin to temporarily disable him.

Any defense against this hold must be performed with force and very quickly before the hold is fully applied. The fact is, once this hold is applied correctly, it is seldom possible to escape from it before unconsciousness ensues. The hold's effectiveness is one of the main reasons why we teach this in all of our law-enforcement training.

Scenario: *The attacker begins to apply a rear naked stranglehold.*

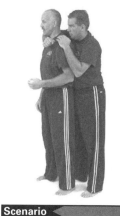

Scenario

Strategy: Obtain release, incapacitate the attacker and leave the scene.

Tactics:

1-2 As the attacker slides his forearm around your neck from behind, try to force your chin downward and shrug your shoulders upward hard so that his arm cannot encircle your throat. Using the hand on the same side as the attacker's arm, grab his encircling wrist and try to clamp it to your chest as you simultaneously drive the elbow of your other arm backwards into his torso.

Continued on page 76.

1-2

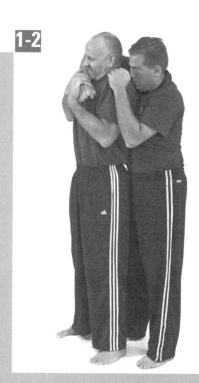

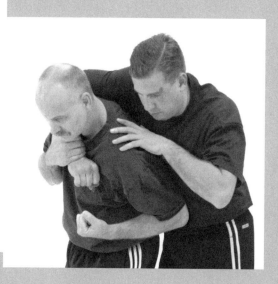

3 Changing hands, maintain the grip on his wrist, immediately duck forward and twist underneath, raising your other arm to point straight upward (I call this the John Travolta technique). Raising the arm like this helps to twist the attacker's elbow upward, thus facilitating the escape.

4–5 The defender's free hand is now in the right position for the counterstrike to the Gb.20 point to the rear of the attacker's head. This should stun him.

6 If the attacker is still conscious, you can continue by driving a knee or shin strike into his face.

Leave the scene.

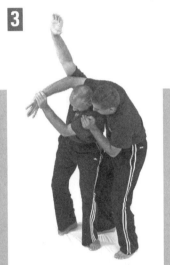

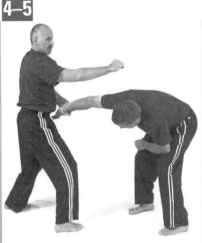

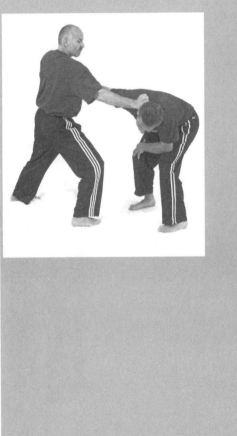

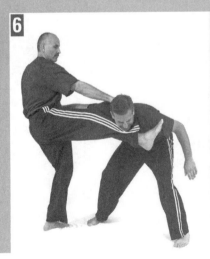

Scenario: You are on your back and the attacker is straddling you in the mounted position, attempting to strangle or punch you.

Strategy: Avoid the strangle, gain release from the hold-down and regain a standing position.

Tactics:

1-3 Press your face firmly into the attacker's lower abdomen while wrapping both of your hands around his hips and pulling hard. Simultaneously make a bridge or thrust up hard with one knee, pinching hard into the flesh on the inside upper thighs as you do so, forcing the attacker to use his hands to prevent himself from being driven over your head and onto his face.

4-5 With the forefinger and thumb of one hand, pinch the vulnerable underside of one of the attacker's upper arms, while further arching and twisting your body to the other side. The reflexive withdrawal reaction to the pinch will cause the attacker to snatch that arm away from the pain and make it easier for you to roll him over.

Immediately get to your feet and leave the scene.

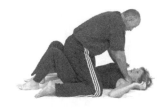

Scenario

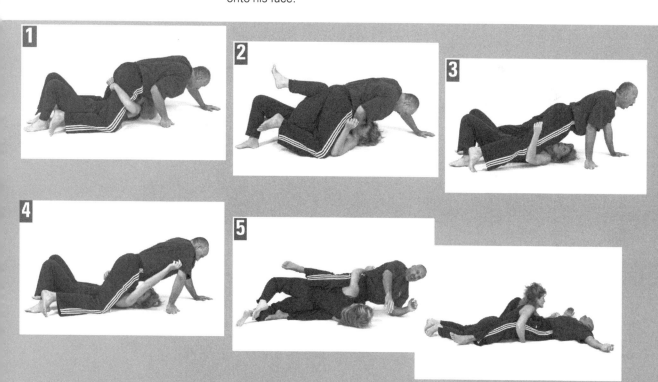

Scenario: You are on your back and the assailant is grappling with you at close range in the mount position.

Strategy: Apply a pressure-point technique to force the attacker to release his grip.

Tactics:

1 Grab hold of the attacker's head and pull it towards your body, thus creating a base for the pressure-point technique.

2 Maintaining a hard grip on the head, place the tip of the thumb of the other hand or the middle joint of that thumb over one of the available pressure points: Tw.17 behind the ear and temple point, Si.18 under the cheek bone. Then drive the thumb hard towards the center of the head, vibrating it as you do so. This continued pressure will create a reflexive dropping action in the attacker, who will release his grip and attempt to pull away.

Scenario

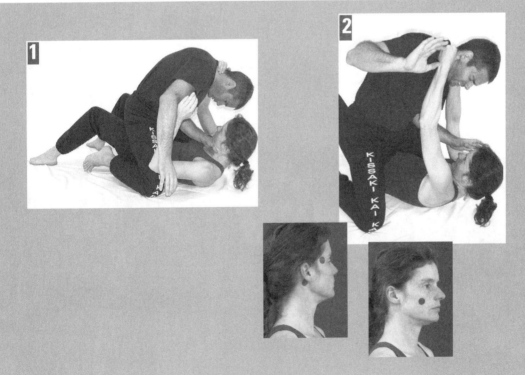

3 As soon as he releases his grip, bridge your body sharply upward and continue to apply hard pressure on whichever point you are using Tw.17.

4 As he is forced in the direction of the pressure, twist your body in the same direction to throw him off you and get up as quickly as you can.

5 Either apply a follow-up control technique or simply leave the scene. In this instance strike to Cv.22.

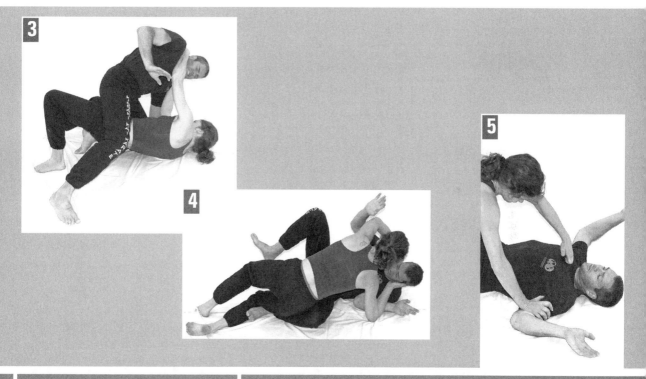

Variation: This technique is also effective if the attacker is between your legs in an attempted rape position.

In this situation, other alternative defenses using the vital points are possible. For example, you might attack the assailant's eyes with finger jabs. Pinches can be applied to the spleen meridian on the inner thigh. The nipples are extremely sensitive to pinching and twisting attacks. Frequently using these minor pressure-point applications will allow you to escalate the defense by then perhaps grabbing and twisting fingers as an aid to escape.

Technique 1: Bilateral vascular neck restraint

In the old Chinese systems of Chin Na and Dim Mak, the technique of causing unconsciousness by this method was called "sealing the blood." It is a technique I have taught to law-enforcement agencies all over the world to great effect, as it has no recorded history of deleterious repercussions. Despite this fact, some police departments will not allow this technique to be used at all. This is unfortunate because in certain instances, such as when a perpetrator is under the influence of PCP or other hugely stimulating drugs, the technique is one of few that can be used to subdue him safely.

Scenario: *You are attempting to restrain and control a violent attacker from the rear.*

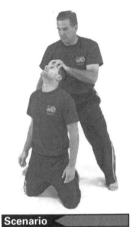

Strategy: Temporarily stun or cause the perpetrator to lose consciousness in order for handcuffs or restraints to be applied.

Tactics:

1 Pull the perpetrator's head backwards with one hand while simultaneously sliding your other arm around his neck until the hollow of your elbow is over the front of his throat

Scenario

2 Once your arm is in place, thrust the perpetrator's head forward again while gripping your forearm with the hand of the arm applying the choke. The perpetrator's head is kept levered forward as the arms now squeeze together, creating a strong inward pressure on either side of the carotid arteries and jugular veins.

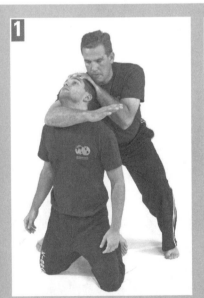

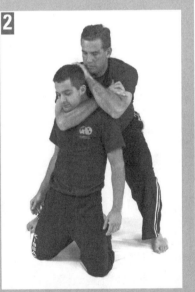

The action is to block the flow of freshly oxygenated blood into the brain while preventing the exit of deoxygenated blood. The brain needs oxygen in order to function but this technique creates a pool of deoxygenated blood dammed up in the brain. Therefore the brain loses consciousness. The pressure on the carotid sinuses at the side of the neck triggers the baroreceptors, which measure blood pressure as well as affect the vagus nerve, which has an effect on heart rate. The result is a slowing of the circulation, which, in addition to the lack of oxygen in the brain, brings about unconsciousness; the carotid sinus cannot distinguish between a physical abnormality or the effect of a blow or external pressure. Interestingly, these are the very factors that make the technique relatively safe: once unconsciousness ensues, the same carotid sinus activity will create a reaction of increasing the heart rate and blood pressure, which will aid recovery.

Defensive Techniques
Headbutt

It is surprising just how often in a defensive scenario it is possible to use the headbutt. In many classes I get an adverse reaction from students who are not used to considering the head as a weapon. In fact it is a very good one, weighing between an eighth and a tenth of one's body weight. Being struck by a correctly delivered headbutt is similar to being hit by a bowling ball. In some parts of the world it is considered a weapon of choice; in Glasgow, Scotland, for example, it is known as "the Glasgow kiss."

It is important to strike with the upper part of the forehead (so that the nose remains untouched) or the back of the head. Any blow striking the attacker's chin, nose, cheek or eyebrow ridge will have a great effect.

Tactics:

A When the attacker is in front, remember to tuck your chin in and drop your head forward—you do not want your nose or eyebrow ridges to come into contact with the hard bone of the assailant's skull.

B When an opponent is to your rear, snap the head backwards a number of times into the assailant's face.

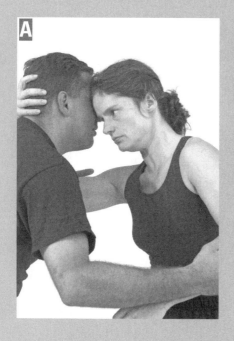

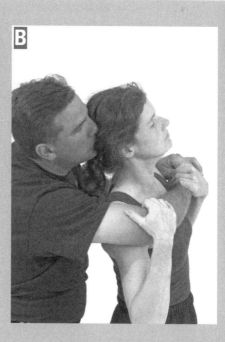

Female Prison Officer Saved from Violent Attack

The following letter received from a training instructor demonstrates conclusively just how effective a weapon the headbutt can be.

It's Wednesday morning after my Tuesday-night class. This gave me a chance to get some more details on the incident at the prison where your techniques were used to save a female employee. As in many second-hand war stories, some exaggerations took place but the central truth remained. In all cases of assault, formal reports are made and reported to the staff. It turns out that the prisoner was not 6' 7" and close to 400 pounds ("huge") as the second-hand reports described him. But he was 6' 4" and 330 pounds—still rather "huge" compared to the female supervisor he assaulted, who was only 5' 7".

It turns out that she had seen your video, and on the basis of that one viewing used your basic short-range knife defense in which the attacker's right arm is blocked and tucked under her arm. She then attempted a headbutt and may have made some contact, but when the attacker moved his head away, she butted hard again, this time landing her strike on his collarbone, where it connects to the shoulder. The collarbone broke.

She then used her right knee to strike the attacker in the groin—a nice touch—and threw (or more probably) rolled him to the ground using the arm she still had tucked away in her armpit. He probably landed on his right shoulder with the broken collarbone—and the battle was over.

After this more-detailed description based on the incident report, I asked my student (the 6'5" prison guard) the critical question, "What part of the female supervisor's actions were also part of the training given at the prison?" His answer was short and sweet: "None!"

So there is "the rest of the story," and even more congratulations are in order since the arm trap set up the headbutt and the groin strike and started the otherwise defenseless young lady on the path out of her horrifying and quite possibly fatal encounter.

Dr. R.S.L, safety instructor

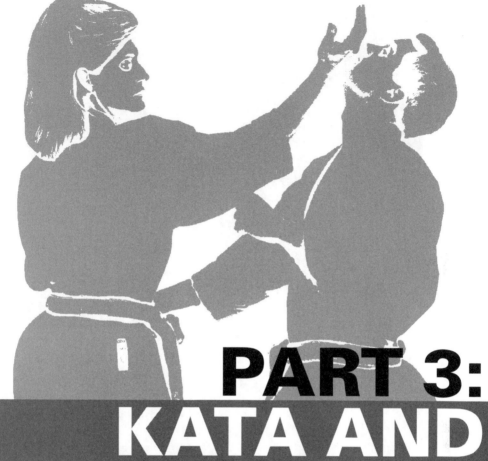

PART 3:
KATA AND APPLICATIONS

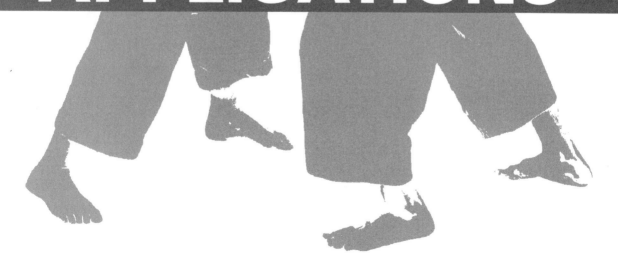

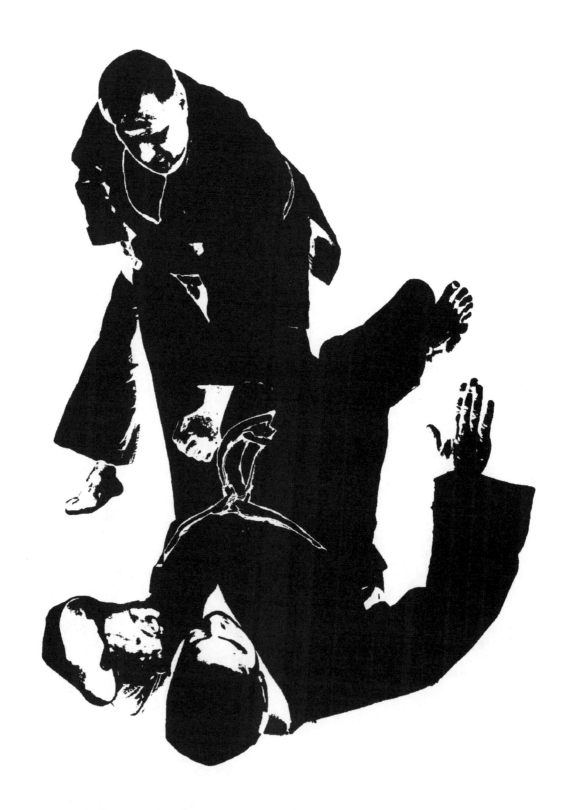

THE IMPORTANCE
OF KATA

A *kata* is a series of defensive, martial techniques performed against a succession of imaginary assailants, taking a minute or two to complete. All the defensive techniques shown earlier in the book are derived directly or indirectly from kata. However, you should be able to carry out these techniques effectively without any knowledge of their origins. Why, then, are kata considered to be so important?

For one thing, not everybody is the same. We all have different body types. Some people are tall, some are short. Some are heavily muscled, some are slight of stature; some are heavy, some are light. Then there are different personality types—some people are aggressive, some are passive; some move quickly, some move more slowly. All these factors help determine which particular type of defensive technique best suits each individual.

Although there are only so many ways to kick or punch, self-defense is not a "one size fits all" situation. The various kata are a compendium of the great diversity of ways to achieve the same objectives. Only by having knowledge of a number of these kata will the student come to learn which particular type of *waza* ("technique") will best suit him or her. What works effectively for a strong six-foot athlete will not necessarily be the technique of choice for a much smaller, lighter individual.

Naturally, having the knowledge of pressure-point fighting will go a long way towards evening up the odds, and generally towards weighting them in favor of the defender. Nonetheless, simply possessing knowledge without the skills to apply it is as useless as learning to read music, but not being able to play an instrument—great as an academic exercise, but useless at a party!

The old masters knew the value of kata and they exist in most of the classical martial arts. Not understanding them, on the other hand, has led to their use in most post–World War II karate as calisthenic training aids. By comprehending kata's correct purpose as the physical encyclopedia of martial principles, each student can find a method of executing defensive techniques that properly suits his or her own physical type.

Modern athletic training makes great use of mental rehearsal in order to master a physical skill. Sitting quietly and running an imaginary scenario through one's mind, concentrating on a successful outcome, is also a very effective way to train self-defense techniques. Imagining the confrontation and the successful reaction to it helps to make the scenario less frightening should it ever really happen because it will not be a completely unknown situation. It is fear of the unknown that has the most disadvantageous effect on a person.

By performing the techniques from the kata in the mind, then physically while still imagining the reality of the attack scenario that had been previously visualized, the body and mind get used to the situation and will react more quickly to it in reality, should it ever be necessary. This is a significant factor because, to be effective, one must train as close to reality as is safely possible; every serious student should include visualization training in their program.

The kata should be performed with great intensity, concentrating on keeping an image of the attack scenario and the assailant uppermost in the mind. In this fashion, the kata are also excellent training aids when there is no partner available to train with.

So, in brief, the kata are valuable physical dictionaries of defensive techniques geared to a variety of body types. They can be used to sharpen technique by both mentally and physically rehearsing the attack and defense scenarios they comprise and they can help to direct the student to more techniques of the kind that best suit their individual requirements.

The Correct Use of Kata

The Japanese martial arts have a long history of committing techniques, especially those peculiar to their particular system, either to paper in the form of *makimono* ("scrolls") or to physical patterns of movement (the kata). Invariably, these scrolls were treasured and kept highly secret, the knowledge contained only made fully available to those who were immediate family members, or who had mastered the training syllabus over years of study and practice.

In much the same way, the physical collections of the principles upon which the particular *ryu* ("school") founded its training in combat were also kept secret, but in a somewhat different fashion. Just like a written scroll could be interpreted by anyone who managed to get hold of a copy, the physical techniques of a kata could be learned. However, the inner meaning of the principles exemplified by those techniques were not immediately observable.

The karate kata were originally passed on by oral tradition, the only apparent exception being a collection of strategy tactics and *waza* from the White Crane kempo tradition, known as the "Bubishi." Over the years, this has led to much confusion in regards to the value that should be placed upon the kata and the usefulness in learning defensive methods. That this confusion existed for so long is testimony to the obfuscation employed by the old masters, who were not at all happy to share the inner secrets of what made their schools so effective.

At least one old master, consulted by Yoshitake Funakoshi (son of Master Gichin Funakoshi), admitted that because he had been pestered so much by another martial arts teacher he eventually agreed to show him the movements of his kata. But, he proudly admitted, "I showed him all the wrong *bunkai*!" (*Bunkai* is the application of the techniques.) This anecdote can be found in the book *Karate-Do Nyumon*. The very fact that this happened shows without a doubt that it is possible to teach a seemingly effective physical technique, while at the heart lies another reality altogether that is not perceivable at surface level.

The problem that arises from a basic (and often deliberately created) misunderstanding of karate kata is that it then becomes impossible to practice the kata correctly. Unlike judo kata, which is practiced in pairs and the *waza* is more immediately evident, karate kata is for the most part practiced by single individuals. The perceived meanings (*omote waza*) tend to mirror the physical outward form of the techniques in the sequence, and appear to have obvious applications: a punch is a punch, a block is a block, etc. However, the school may well have had secret meanings disguised within the obvious outward form. These are the *okuden* or *ura waza*—the dangerously effective hidden techniques of throwing, striking, choking and joint manipulation

No *ryu* wanted its competitors, and perhaps its enemies, to know its secrets; by deliberately maintaining the policy of only revealing these secrets to its inner core of long-term students, and by only disclosing the outward *omote* meanings, the true principles of combat remained hidden. (Of course, this naturally served to keep the secrets from latter generations of Western students, too.)

With the defeat of the Japanese in World War II and the occupation of Okinawa, American servicemen first became exposed to the art of karate. In the main, these were tough individuals accustomed to the discipline and rigors of military life and the direct use of force in gaining victory. They were also generally unable to speak Hogen (the Okinawa dialect) or much Japanese. Teaching, therefore, was mainly done using a "monkey see, monkey do" approach, with the greater part of any subtlety completely lost. The outward form, the *omote*, was learned and thus began the whole train of events that introduced karate to the West.

Later, when the Japanese began exporting their forms of the now-altered Okinawan fighting art, they concentrated upon sending forth strong, dynamic and forceful instructors who could more than hold their own in face-to-face encounters. Given that what was now taught in Japan was itself a weakened sport form of the original, and that by far the greater part of just a few years of training was spent in honing powerful combat skills within the sporting framework of rules and objectives, it is not surprising that these Japanese instructors themselves knew little, if anything at all, about the real secrets of karate.

Some 30 years ago, I remember that any attempt to question our Japanese instructors was met with admonitions to "Just train harder!" Thinking and questioning were not on the agenda. The practice of kata certainly had a big place in the training regime, but it was there to teach balance and coordination, concentration and stamina. At no time were any of the techniques given anything other than a cursory glance as being useful for actual combat. The few occasions in which the *bunkai* were demonstrated only served to show their uselessness in anything other than a carefully scripted situation. These demonstrations involved a defender surrounded by four attackers who had predetermined roles. They'd attack the defender one by one, allowing him time to deliver exaggerated techniques before addressing the next attack. Never were the attackers allowed to attack all at once. This meaningless ritual is carried out to this day even in dojos in Japan and Okinawa.

The material written by many masters, including Funakoshi and Itosu, continually emphasizes that kata were the foundation and very bedrock of karate and that they should be correctly understood and practiced in a serious and determined manner against imaginary attackers, almost as if one were on a battlefield. Given that the very nature of karate in the West was formulated upon the teachings of those who had not fully understood the complexities of the art, it is not surprising that the remarks of the early masters were somewhat incomprehensible to modern students.

At this juncture, it will be beneficial to consider the thoughts of one of the greatest early masters, Kenwa Mabuni, the founder of the Shito-Ryu karate school and one of the first to introduce the Okinawan art into

Japan. Mabuni was said to have known just about all the kata in Okinawa; if anyone needed to check a move or polish a kata, then it was to Mabuni that they turned. Mabuni at one period also worked as a police officer, so it is quite credible that he would have been in a position to test the effectiveness of some of his knowledge. He is also known to have accepted challenges in the street from time to time.

In 1934, for a publication called *Karate Kenkyu* ("Karate Research"), Mabuni wrote an essay titled "Kata wa tadashiku renshu seyo" ("Practice kata correctly") that made a number of important statements about the value and function of kata.

> *"In karate, the most important thing is kata. Into the kata of karate are woven every manner of attack and defense technique. Therefore kata must be practiced properly, with a good understanding of their* bunkai *meaning."* Unfortunately, since most of the kata being taught was surface level only, a *"good understanding of their* bunkai*"* was impossible. Mabuni continued, *"There may be those who neglect the practice of kata, thinking that it is sufficient to just practice* kumite *[sparring—probably pre-arranged sparring] that has been created based upon their knowledge of the kata, but that will never lead to true advancement."*

Mabuni went on to explain that the techniques of karate have innumerable possibilities and variations, so that it would be impossible to construct predetermined *kumite* to reflect this. However, "If one sufficiently and regularly practices kata correctly, it will serve as a foundation for performing—when a crucial time comes—any of the innumerable variations."

Mabuni was well aware that on their own, kata were not the whole answer, as he pointed out the necessity of studying things like correct combat distancing, correct body movement, *kumite* and conditioning. However, he also added that simply amassing a large number of kata with little understanding of the depth of them is a useless exercise: "Breadth, no matter how great, means little without depth….If you sufficiently study two or three kata as your own and strive to perform them correctly, when the need arises, that training will spontaneously take over and will be shown to be surprisingly effective." He emphasized that it doesn't matter how much time and effort you devote to sparring and striking the makiwara ("traditional striking post"), because if your kata training is incorrect, you will find that when the moment comes to use your skills, you will probably fail.

The essential conclusion of this essay is quite simple and direct: The most important thing for anyone training in karate is to practice kata correctly, and one of the most important features of this is to understand their meaning. This advice has been more or less ignored over the years, with hardly any real attempts being made to encourage a proper understanding of the secrets of the kata.

Learning from the Original Blueprints

For one reason or another—the urge to secrecy, lack of knowledge, forgetfulness—the essence of the inner meanings of the *bunkai* were not passed on to the younger Japanese karate-*ka*, and in turn were never passed on to their students in the West. I began my own research into the real meaning of the kata in the 1970s. My first publications attracted some attention, not a little of which was derogatory and dismissive. I likened the kata to dictionaries, with each word (technique) having numerous meanings (possible applications). I equated the endless repetition of basics and mindless kata to a child's repetition of the alphabet—vital, but of no use at all unless superseded. Basic *waza* must build effective combat response just as the letters of the alphabet should be made into words, prose and poetry.

To correctly understand the original intentions of the deviser, originator or compiler of the individual kata, it is necessary to research the earliest forms of that kata. This is not always an easy task, as many have been changed intentionally; for example, Master Itosu's original Pinan kata were deliberately altered to formulate the Heian kata. At the same time, other changes were effected: the front snap kick became a side snap kick, the *neko ashi dachi* (cat foot stance) became the *ko kutsu dachi* (back foot stance).

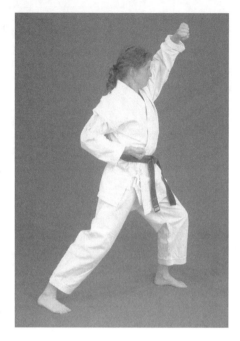

These changes are fairly obvious, however. Over the generations, with no real intention at all, sometimes variations are introduced and become adopted. Some might occur because a mistake has been made, while others take place because it is felt that a genuine improvement can be made. I recall at one time Master Kanazawa introducing the *jodan mawashi geri* (upper roundhouse kick) into the kata Empi, on the basis that the kick does not appear in any of the kata and could well fit into this one. After a few years, this practice was quietly dropped.

Masters do make mistakes, and students do perpetuate them. For this reason, it is often impossible to get back to the very earliest example—the source, so to speak. Fortunately, my early experiences researching and translating Old Icelandic saga and Old English texts provided me with the means to evaluate, discriminate and arrive at probable conclusions by examining and comparing a host of sources. In addition, I devised the "Rules of Combat" (an expansion of the very points made by Mabuni above) and researched the use of pressure points in the human body that would prove beneficial in combat.

Eventually I stripped away a whole morass of further obfuscation and arrived at what I believe to be the essence of the kata: the principles of combat allied to powerful techniques utilizing the weaknesses of the human body.

The Significance of Boyd's Law

John (Richard) Boyd (1927–1997) was a U.S. Air Force fighter pilot who gained notoriety as a military strategist. Among other reasons, Boyd is significant in regards to individual combat because of his formulation of the decision cycle, or the OODA loop. The acronym stands for "Observation, Orientation, Decision and Action," which are the processes through which the brain cycles when perceiving and reacting to a given situation. According to this concept, the key to victory is being able to make appropriate decisions more quickly than one's opponent. If all else is equal, the protagonist who arrives at the Action element first will have the advantage.

There are at least two major factors here for the martial artist. First, the situation must be correctly assessed and the aggressor's intentions recognized. In other words, cues and clues have to be read. Second, the last stage—action—must be reached in time to react to the situation.

Dr. Darrell Ross, chairman of the Department of Law Enforcement and Justice Administration at Western Illinois University, meticulously analyzed 86 high-profile police-suspect confrontations about which federal lawsuits, alleging excessive force and civil rights violations, were filed. The 121 officers in the study were male, mostly patrolmen, and from 94 agencies from across the United States. Suspects were killed in 97 percent of these controversial confrontations; all the involved officers survived. Of the ensuing civil suits that went to court (86 percent), all the officers were judged to have acted correctly.

Ross identified certain essential skills these officers brought to their decision making, and he described the type of training he believed best builds these strengths. Under ideal circumstances, decision making is a deliberative process that follows "schematic, sequentially ordered steps," with time to evaluate options, weigh relative risks and potential benefits, and perhaps even to field-test possibilities. In academic circles, this is called the "rational analysis" model.

When faced with lethal-force confrontations, cops rarely have that luxury. In such situations, "There is no 'decision tree,' as in the rational analysis model," Ross wrote. Decisions tend to be made according to a "recognition-primed" model. That is, you quickly "read" what you're dealing with on the basis of certain cues and patterns that seem familiar from past training and experience and you choose a course of action based on what those indicators seem reasonably to be predicting. "The decision may still be rational and logical, but it's not reached through a rational sequence."

A very important factor is having a heightened sense of situational awareness. The officers were keenly attuned to potential danger signals from subjects and from the surrounding environment. The officers were able to correctly anticipate, detect and recognize patterns of behavior, which enabled them to select an appropriate course of action.

They were also effective in perceiving the suspects' body movements, hand actions and other behavior that could signal a pending attack.

The conclusions that Ross drew from the findings once again underline the fundamental importance of correct training: "If you want to achieve proficiency and continue to make progress in a skill, you have to train and practice in an environment where you are required to use that skill."

To develop acute skill in lethal-force decision making and delivery, he suggested the following, based on his findings:

1 Training should be interactive with appropriate environmental and human behavior exhibited and should correctly reflect commonly encountered conditions.

2 Training should be such as to apply sufficient pressure, and should be of a changing nature to demand concentration in the face of distraction and correct selection of appropriate technique. The training should reflect conditions that are to be expected in deadly force encounters.

Training should be frequent. According to Ross, "Training once a year is not a viable mode of learning....You need to keep your mind in a constant state of learning to build expertise. The human brain needs on-going 'upgrades' to keep it fresh and stimulated. Otherwise, it becomes stagnant." In effect, the officers in the study were able to cut through the normal thought processes of everyday situations to correctly appreciate the danger of the actual situation and take rapid action to end it.

Once again we see the importance of directing real martial training towards reality. Each time we rehearse a scenario, we make it easier to recognize its salient features when it actually occurs. This cuts down any cognitive time and allows us to react with tactics that have been practiced time and time again. The OODA loop is thus circumvented by proper training.

Boyd also pointed out the importance of keeping the enemy in the OODA loop by "presenting them with ambiguous, deceptive or novel situations, as well as by operating at a tempo or rhythm they can neither make out nor keep up with." This should be considered as part of the Rules of Combat, discussed earlier. Any means by which one's intentions can be disguised from the assailant will serve to cut down the assailant's ability to react in time.

Thus, when we consider the correct training of kata, we must recognize that (a) It should be as real as possible, therefore the *bunkai* must be correctly understood and practiced not as a solo exercise but with a partner; and (b) practice should reflect reality as closely as possible and training should be repeated frequently.

When combat begins, stress levels will make it extremely difficult for the brain to make conscious, informed decisions. Your reaction should be instant and effective, and based upon the reflexive, conditioned responses you have built by correct training. Each response must be fast—every moment the encounter lasts brings greater danger that something will go wrong. The objective of the *ura* ("hidden") kata *bunkai*, as in the real encounter, is to bring events to a conclusion as fast as is humanly possible.

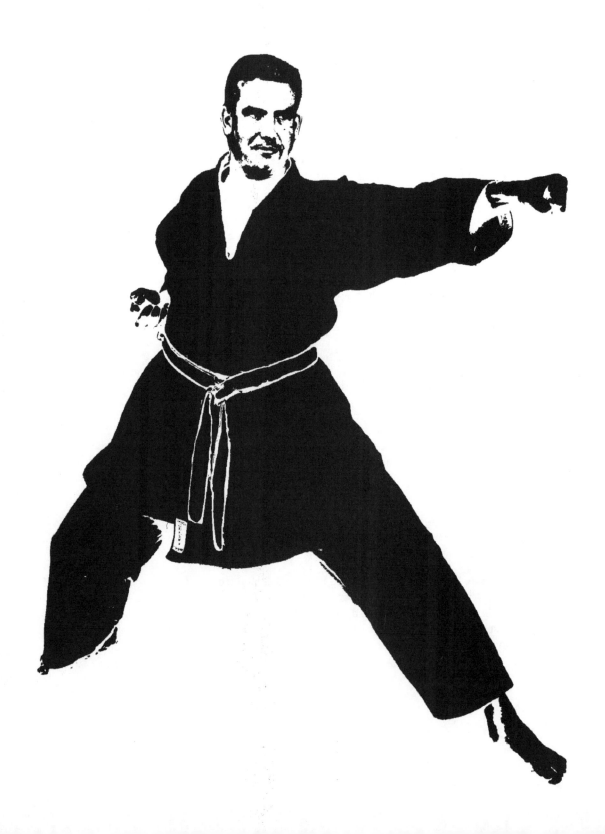

KATA BUNKAI
AND PRESSURE POINTS

This section provides a variety of scenarios and includes their kata origins, which will be enlightening to those who have studied karate, taekwondo and other similar arts. (As my formative years were spent in a Shotokan *dojo*, my examples are mainly from Shotokan kata, but the techniques and principles can be used in any of the defensive systems.)

There is no need to know any of the kata presented in the following section. The photographs show the specific techniques from the kata and the *bunkai* is given to demonstrate the meaning.

By indicating the kata origins, you can trace the principles upon which the technique was founded and understand that it has a long history—hundreds of years, in some cases—of successful use in combat. Naturally, no one ever constructed a kata using techniques that failed. Bear in mind, however, that some of the old masters deliberately obscured the real meanings of the moves, as they considered them too dangerous to reveal to potential enemies or rivals.

Knowing that the techniques are tried and tested—not "pulled out of the air"—you can have confidence in them. A large number of them, in fact, have been incorporated into the law-enforcement and Special Forces training that we teach around the world. Remember, however, that these are certainly not the only *bunkai* for the particular technique. In real combat, one does not want to select from 50 responses in order to deal with 20 different attacks. The best thing is to have a Swiss Army knife of perhaps six or eight *bunkai* that deal with the 20 attacks.

If you spend some time mastering these techniques, you'll have the added bonus of knowing their origins, which will allow you to make further progress by seeking out the other techniques in the same kata.

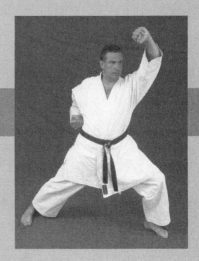

Age uke
upward block

There are many techniques that occur frequently in different kata, signifying their usefulness once the bunkai is understood. The upward block (*age uke*) is one such technique. It can indeed be a block, but it is much more effective as an arm lock or forearm strike.

Scenario: The assailant seizes you by one lapel and attempts to strike you in the face.

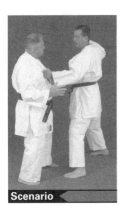

Scenario

Strategy: Use a distraction technique to prevent the blow to the face from landing, temporarily disable the attacker and leave the scene.

Tactics:

1-2 Simultaneously make a distraction technique with one hand while pressing the attacker's gripping hand firmly to your body. As you do this, move your body away from the attacker's striking hand. The assailant will react by drawing back reflexively from the distraction technique and his gripping arm will straighten, revealing the Lu.5 point that is the target of the next defensive strike.

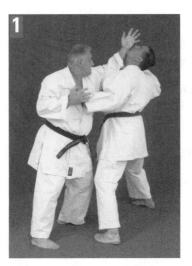

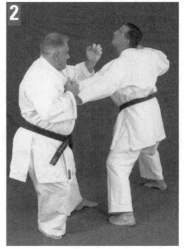

3-4 Drive your forearm down hard through the Lu.5 point. This will immediately snap the attacker's head forward into the upward forearm strike (the *age uke*) to the St.5 point on the side of his jaw for a stun or full knockout, depending on the force of the blow. (The technique is executed with speed and by introducing the extra impact gained by adding body weight as you slide away and then back in, it becomes very powerful and can easily cause a full knockout.)

Note: The primary target is the Lu.5 point on the side of the jaw, but equally effective results can be achieved by striking any of the points at the side of the neck.

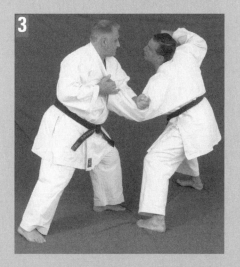

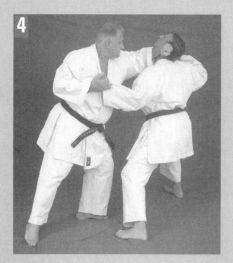

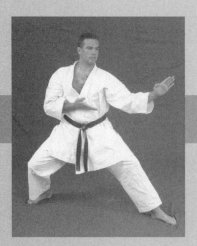

Shuto uke
knifehand block

Again, this technique occurs frequently in different kata, signifying its usefulness once the *bunkai* is understood. Most karateka underestimate the use of the front hand in this technique and place their emphasis upon the perceived weapon, the "blocking" hand.

In many years of *kumite* ("sparring") or in real situations, I have never seen this technique used at all, and the reason is that—as commonly taught—it will not work, and everyone knows that. If used correctly however, it is an essential weapon and its occurrence in a wide number of kata testifies to this.

When applying the technique correctly, the hand that goes to the front first and is then snapped back is of primary importance, as this is, in fact, the blocking hand, used to deflect an incoming blow. The perceived "knifehand block" is an immediate follow-up, delivered with power to one of the vulnerable areas on the attacker's arm, head or neck.

There are many techniques that occur frequently in different kata, signifying their usefulness once the bunkai is understood. The upward block (*age uke*) is one such technique. It can indeed be a block, but it is much more effective as an arm lock or forearm strike.

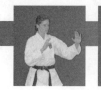

Knifehand Block

Scenario: The assailant throws a left straight jab punch to your face or attempts to grab with both hands.

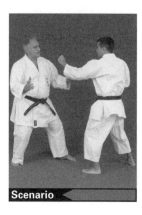

Scenario

Strategy: Stop the blow from making contact, temporarily disable the attacker and leave the scene.

Tactics:

1-2 As the blow is delivered, deflect it with the open palm of your right hand while simultaneously shifting to the outside of the attacker's centerline and preparing your left hand to strike

3 As the attacker is unbalanced, slide forward and strike hard, in a downward direction with the outside edge of the left knifehand, aiming at the Lu.5 point on the attacker's forearm. This will further unbalance him.

Continued on page 98.

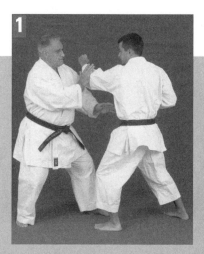

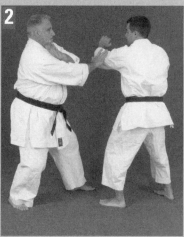

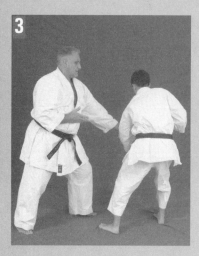

4 Immediately step forward so that your right leg goes behind your opponent's legs and drive your right knifehand hard downward into his face or neck. As you strike, grasp the attacker's punching arm with your left hand, which delivered the initial blow.

5 Complete the move by slamming your whole body into him as you deliver the final head or neck strike. This will drive the attacker down to the ground.

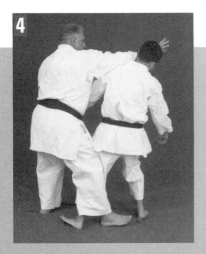

In most kata, *shuto uke* is performed in pairs. The reason for this is shown here.

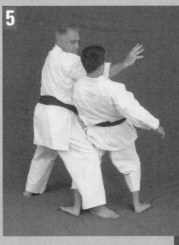

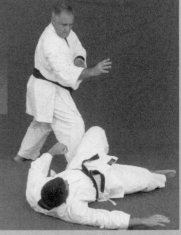

Nagashi uke, teisho, manji gamae
sweeping block, palm heel, high-low arm

Once again, this technique or a variation of it occurs in many different kata. It is extremely useful in close-range grappling situations, or when the attacker attempts to kick you.

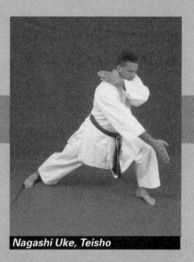

Nagashi Uke, Teisho

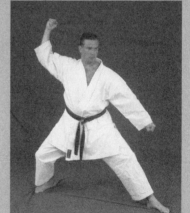

Manji Gamae

Sweeping Block, Palm Heel, High-low Arm

Scenario 1: *The attacker closes in on you in an attempt to grapple.*

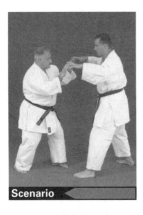

Scenario

Strategy: Prevent the grappling attack, force the assailant to the ground and leave the scene.

Tactics:

1 Assume a defensive position with your chin down, knees in and hands up.

2-3 As the assailant attempts to close and grapple, deliver a sharp back-hand strike to his nose, withdrawing the hand immediately to the side of your head. This will force a reflexive withdrawal response.

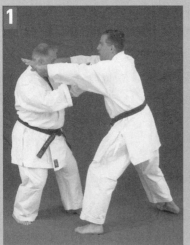

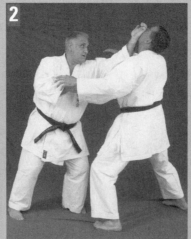

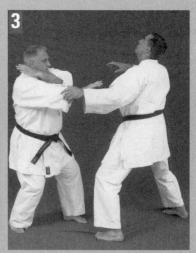

4 Immediately drop down and drive the elbow of the same arm downward into the opponent's lower abdomen while simultaneously seizing his ankle with your other hand.

5-6 As you drive the elbow strike through the attacker's torso, yank his foot towards you and stand up. If necessary, disable the attacker with a punch to the exposed groin.

Leave the scene.

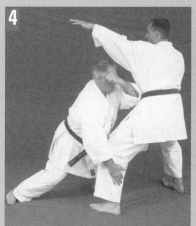
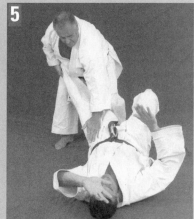
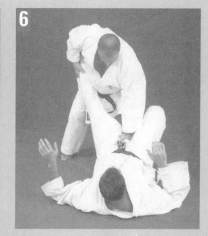

Variation: If necessary, you can aid the application of the throw by changing the elbow strike (after it has been delivered) into a simple pushing technique. The attacker will be thrown onto his back.

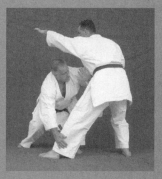
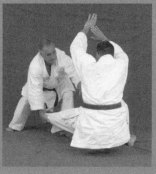
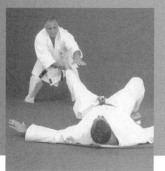

Scenario 2: *The attacker attempts to kick you with his right foot.*

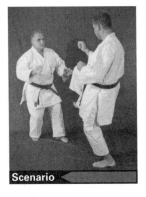

Scenario

Strategy: Prevent the kick from landing, force the assailant to the ground and leave the scene.

Tactics:

1 As the kick comes towards you, use the same-side forearm to deflect it towards the attacker's centerline.

2 Immediately drop your body weight and catch the kicking leg in the crook of your right arm.

3 Shift your body 45 degrees towards the attacker's centerline and drive your left elbow, fist or forearm hard downward through the Sp.11 point on the inside of the thigh of the kicking leg. This combined action will buckle his leg outward and force him to the ground.

Leave the scene.

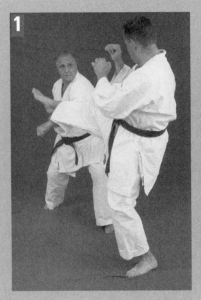

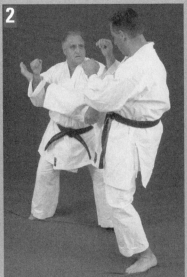

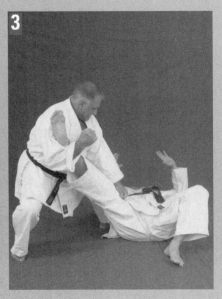

Haiwan uke, ura zuki, tetsui
double-hand block, "knuckles down" punch, hammerfist strike

One of the most important skills to develop is the ability to have your hands do more than one thing at a time. Used in conjunction with pre-determined responses from striking vital points (knowing ahead of time where your attacker's body will be), having your hands ready in a predetermined, optimum position makes the delivery of your counter-strikes much faster. This particular *bunkai* is an ideal example.

To show the versatility of correctly understanding the principles within the kata, three sequences utilizing the same *bunkai* are given below. The same principles are being used in each case: using both hands simulta-neously, attacking high and low, never allowing the attacker to deliver a blow or finish an attack, ensuring correct body positioning and using the vital points. All this—contained within more or less the same defensive paradigm to defend against different attacks—shows the value of fol-lowing the advice of the old masters: to really understand the kata and *bunkai* correctly!

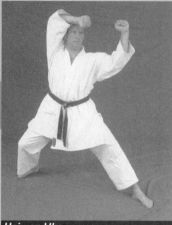

Haiwan Uke

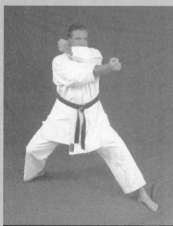

Ura Zuki

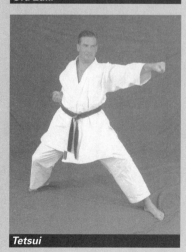

Tetsui

Double-hand Block, "Knuckles Down" Punch, Hammerfist Strike

Scenario 1: *The attacker grips your left wrist with his left hand and prepares to strike you with his right.*

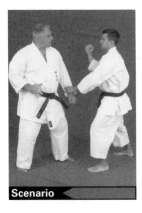

Scenario

Strategy: Prevent the blow from landing, temporarily disable the attacker and leave the scene.

Tactics:

1 The instant your wrist is grabbed, move sharply 45 degrees to the outside of the attacker's centerline to evade a potential strike. Simultaneously raise your gripped arm to head height, pulling it close to your face. This will turn the attacker's arm to expose the Tw.12 point in the triceps muscle.

2 Immediately smash your right hammerfist into the TW point to unbalance the attacker and turn his head to expose the Gb.20 point.

3 With your left hand, deliver a hard hammer strike to the exposed Gb. point to stun the attacker or render him unconscious.

Leave the scene.

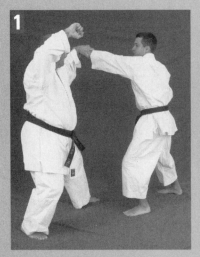

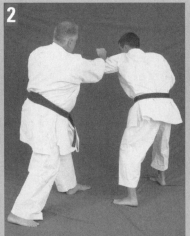

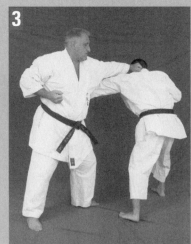

Scenario 2: The attacker assumes a boxing stance and prepares to throw a left jab at your face.

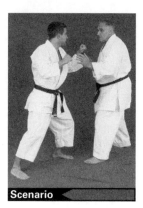

Scenario

Strategy: Prevent the blow from landing, temporarily disable the attacker and leave the scene.

Tactics:

1 Immediately slide forward (the attacker will not expect this) and deflect the punch with your left forearm while raising your right hand to the side of your face. Your right hand continues to push his punching arm outward.

2 Without stopping, drive a left backfist to the Gv.26 point under his nose. This will invoke a reflexive withdrawal response to make the assailant momentarily halt the attack and jerk his head backwards. (In fact, the same response will be invoked by simply driving your backfist hard into his nose.)

3-4 As he pulls his head backwards, his torso will be exposed: Drive a right uppercut ("knuckles-down" punch) into the Gb.24 point on his rib cage. This will turn him slightly sideways and jerk his head forward again, directly into the knockout blow, which is a left hammerfist strike to the Gb.20 point at the back of his head.

Leave the scene.

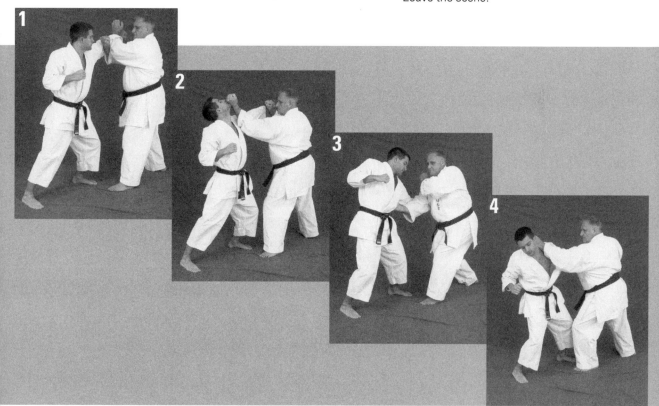

Scenario 3: *The attacker seizes your shoulder from behind with his left hand in an attempt to turn you around or detain you.*

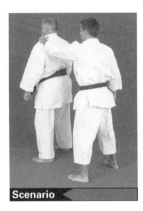

Scenario

Strategy: Maintain your balance, gain release from the grip, temporarily incapacitate the assailant and leave the scene.

Tactics:

1 Raising both arms, immediately twist in a counterclockwise direction and step outward 45 degrees until you are facing the attacker.

2 As you turn, make sure that your front (left) hand is raised high enough so that your elbow can travel freely over his extended gripping arm. Immediately deliver a hard backfist strike to anywhere on his face. This will cause him to reflexively jerk away from the blow, exposing his torso.

3 Simultaneously drive an uppercut with your right fist into the Gb.24 point on the ribcage, while withdrawing your left hand in preparation for the coup de grace. The blow to the Gb.24 point will cause the attacker to bend forward and turn slightly, exposing the Gb.20 point on the back of his head.

4 Immediately strike the Gb.20 point on the back of his head hard with a left hammerfist strike to knock him unconscious.

Leave the scene.

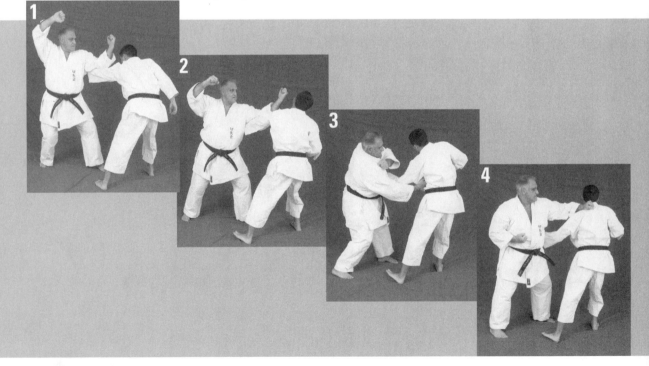

Tekki Shodan/Naihanchi

One of the characteristics of this kata lies in the speed and brutality of its *bunkai*. Unlike practically all other karate kata, which have a pattern allowing the defender to move fairly freely, this kata restricts the defender to a simple side-stepping movement pattern. This appears to be a characteristic of techniques that are not simply self-defensive, but are instrumental in preventing an attack on a third party, which naturally constrains the defender's freedom of movement while demanding extremely effective techniques.

The techniques described here are not the only ones possible; they simply represent some of the principles.

Opening sequence: *Yoi (ready), te uke (hand block), haishu-uchi (backhand strike)*
Scenario: *The attacker moves forward, reaching with an arm either to grab, push or strike.*

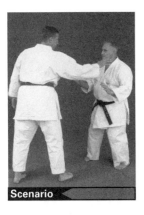

Scenario

Tactics:

1 Simultaneously move into the path of the arm while striking it out to one side with the same-side arm (e.g., use your left if he attacks with his left).

2-3 Now immediately reverse the strike, slamming the back of your hand into the side of the attacker's face, or your forearm into the points on the side of the attacker's neck. This, if done correctly, will stun the attacker and probably drop him to his knees.

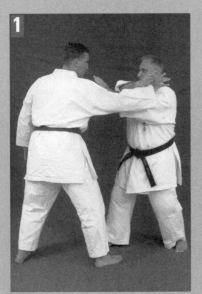

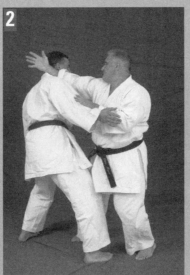

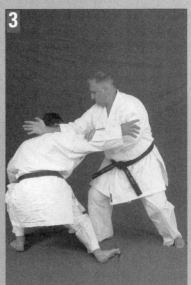

Following three moves: *Empi (elbow), morote koshi gamae (cup and saucer), gedan barai (down block)*
Scenario: *The previous technique has not completely stunned the attacker, who must be finished off.*

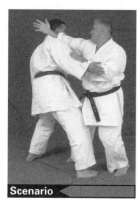
Scenario

Tactics:

1-2 Strike the Gb.20 point on the back of the attacker's head with an elbow strike and immediately seize the head with both hands.

3-5 Jerk his head down to waist level before twisting sharply into a neck throw.

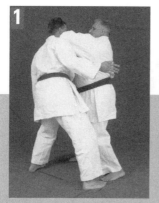

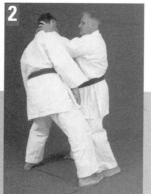

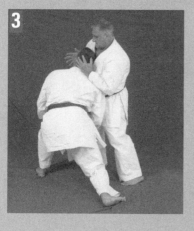

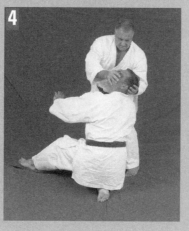

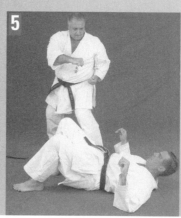

Nami-Gaeshi (Returning Wave Kick)

This is a signature technique of this kata and three of my students have each broken the thigh bone of an attacker when having occasion to use it. Although it occurs four times in the kata, it is such a useful technique that it is possible to incorporate it into almost every defensive sequence. For example, the kick can be added to the previous opening sequence after the initial defensive move and before the strike to the head or neck.

Scenario: *The attacker moves forward, reaching with an arm either to grab, push or strike.*

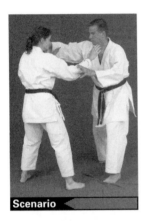

Scenario

Tactics:

1 As you deflect the attacker's arm, twist approximately 45 degrees and snap the heel of your right foot into the attacker's inner thigh (Sp.10). This will unbalance the attacker and cause his head to drop down.

2 Strike with your forearm to the Gb.20 point to effect a knockout.

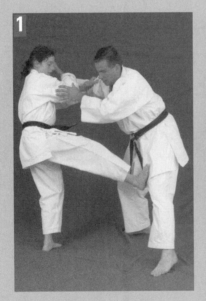
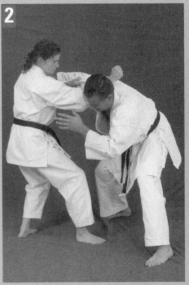

Ura Zuki (Down Block and Uppercut)

Scenario: The attacker seizes your left arm prior to grabbing or striking with his other hand.

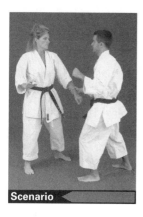

Scenario

Tactics:

1 Immediately use a distraction technique (kick, shout or, as pictured here, backhand to the Gv.26 point).

2 Shift your body away from the attacker's free hand and strike down hard with the bottom of your right forearm onto the Lu.5 point of the attacker's gripping arm. This will reflexively cause the attacker to buckle and drop his head forward.

3 As the strike lands, drive your left fist in an uppercut into the St.5 point on the side of the assailant's jaw to bring about a knockout.

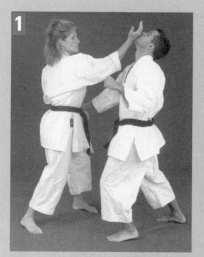

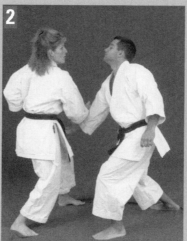

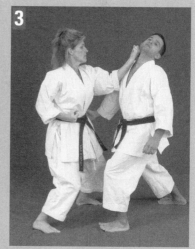

Morote Zuki (Double Punch to Side)

This disguised throwing technique is one of the most effective in the martial arts. It can be employed in a vast number of situations, and one of its great advantages is that neither of the defender's hands has to actually grasp the assailant. Therefore it doesn't matter whether the opponent is clothed or unclothed, wet or covered in sweat or blood. The importance of this throw can be judged by the fact that it occurs in no fewer than three different kata (Tekki, Nijushiho and Jutte), and in a modified form in others.

Scenario: *For example, the throw can be added to the previous sequence after the blow to the St.5 point. The attacker seizes your left arm prior to grabbing or striking with his other hand.*

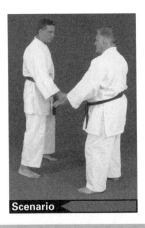

Scenario

Tactics:

1 Immediately use a distraction technique (kick, shout or, as pictured here, backhand to the St.5 point at side of the jaw).

2 Shift your body away from the attacker's free hand and strike down hard with the bottom of your right forearm onto the Lu.5 point of the attacker's gripping arm. This will reflexively cause the attacker to buckle and drop his head forward.

3 As the strike lands, drive your left fist in an uppercut into the St.5 point on the side of the assailant's jaw to bring about a knockout.

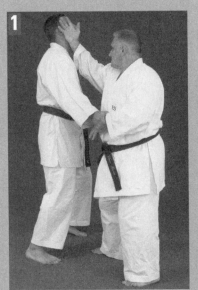

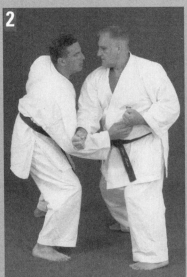

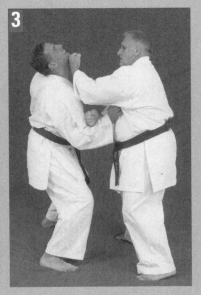

4-6 As the uppercut lands, continue your punch past the attacker's face while stepping your left leg behind the attacker in a violent shoving action, barging the attacker sideways to tumble over your leg. You can make the action more forceful by simultaneously driving your right elbow or forearm backwards into the attacker's face and knock him forcefully to the ground.

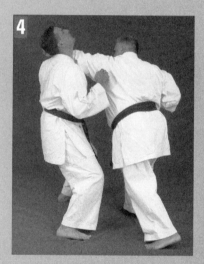

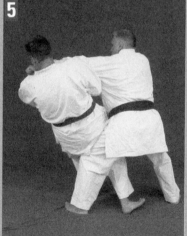

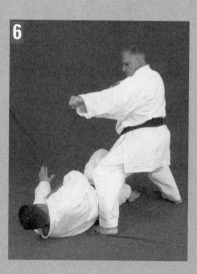

Kanku Dai

Kanku Dai (Kushanku) is considered a seminal kata in Shotokan. There has been a claim that Master Itosu, the creator of Pinan/Heian kata, took certain techniques from Kanku Dai and included them in the new Pinan/Heian kata in a "weakened" form to make the kata safe to be practiced by high school children. This claim is wholly incorrect. There is no difference at all in the performance of the techniques (*waza*). The confusion arose from points we raised earlier in the section "The Correct Use of Kata" in that the hidden (*omote*) knowledge was never passed on with the physical technique.

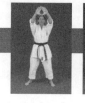

Opening moves: *Both hands, fingertips and thumbs touching, move upwards, part, circle down, shuto uke (knifehand strike).*

Scenario: *The attacker seizes you by the throat with both hands in an attempted strangle.*

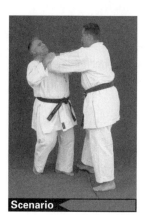

Scenario ◀

Tactics:

1 Immediately thrust the closed fingers of both hands directly into the attacker's eyes or throat Cv.22. This will invoke a flinch withdrawal reflex as the attacker attempts to pull away.

2 Reach up with one hand and grab the attacker's hair, pulling his head sharply down to one side to expose his throat and/or neck.

3 Now drive the edge of your other hand hard down onto the Tw.16, Si.17 or Gb.20 points for a stunning blow.

There are actually a number of very useful, different defensive techniques hidden in this ostensibly simple movement. In one real-life situation, it has saved my head from being struck by an iron bar and it can serve as an opening deflecting or distracting movement for many different follow-up combinations. The value of this technique derives from the fact that it is built upon the normal human reaction to sudden movement, which is to raise both hands quickly in front of the face. It is always an advantage to build a defensive reaction upon a reflex, which the body already possesses.

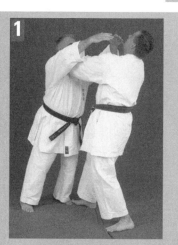

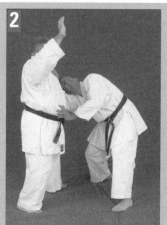

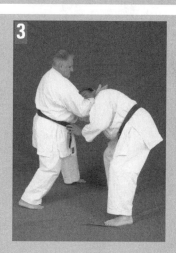

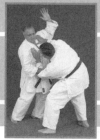

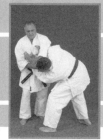

Tip: If the attacker is bald or only has short hair, the technique can be modified by seizing one of his arms and jerking that downward. This will also expose his head or neck for the final strike.

Shuto Uke (Knifehand Block), step forward, Shuto Uke

This technique can be used as described in the previous shuto uke sequence, but in a more serious situation it can be enhanced by delivering a powerful strike to the St.5 point or the Tw.22 point on the side of the head for a knockout.

Scenario: *The attacker punches or attempts to grab you.*

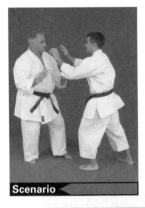

Scenario

Tactics:

1-2 Moving to the outside (position of advantage), palm away the attack and immediately perform a knifehand strike onto the Lu.5 point on the attacker's forearm. This will cause the attacker to jerk forward and downward, exposing his head.

3 Immediately following the knifehand strike to the arm, the attacker will attempt to regain balance. Prepare to deliver a disabling blow to one of the vital points on the face or head.

4 Step forward and immediately drive your other hand or forearm across the attacker's face or neck while sliding your advancing foot behind the attacker's legs. The attacker will be driven to the ground.

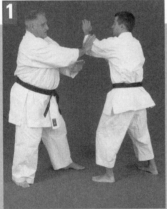
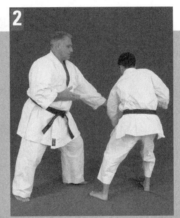
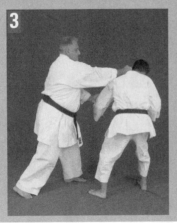
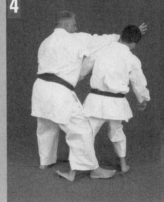
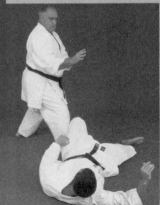

Morote Ura Zuki (Right Augmented Uppercut), Hiza Ate (Knee Smash), throw

Scenario: Attacker attempts to seize you by both lapels or grab you by the throat.

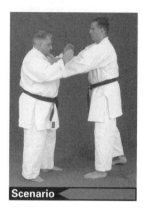

Scenario

Tactics:

1 As the assailant raises both arms, thrust both hands upwards and bring your forearms together hard on the points of the assailant's neck (Si.17, Tw.16). This can be done with both arms together or, more commonly, by stabilizing the head with one hand while driving the forearm of the other arm into the neck.

2 Squeezing hard on the neck, pull the attacker's face hard into your chest and slip the fingers of both hands down to the hypoglossal nerve, running underneath the inside of the chin.

Continued on page 118.

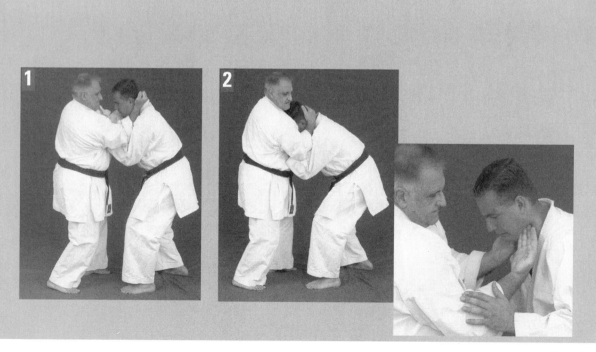

3 Stab upwards hard to invoke a flinch reflex, which will make the attacker abruptly jerk upwards and off balance.

4 Finally, drop down and encircle your arms around both of his knees and barge the attacker with your shoulder or head so that he falls onto his back.

5 If necessary, strike to the exposed groin to disable the attacker.

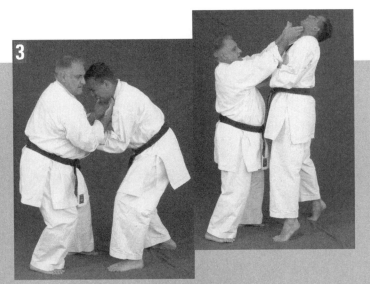

This defense presupposes that the defender initiates the technique before the attacker has obtained a firm hold. If this is not the case, the initial move has to be exchanged for either a double palm strike to the ears or double finger jabs to the eyes. The rest of the technique proceeds as shown.

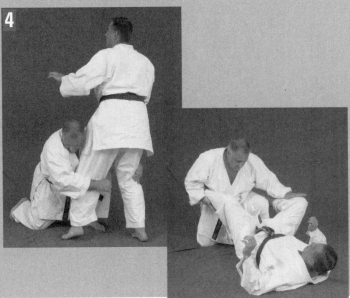

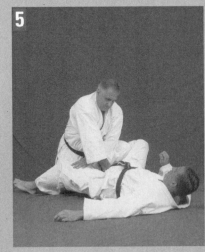

Gyaku Hanmi Shuto Uchi (Knifehand Strike), Mae Geri (Front Kick), Uraken (fist/forearm/elbow)

This sequence demonstrates the depth of the bunkai within the kata. It shows how, with minor adjustments, an attack can be brought to conclusion by driving an opponent to his knees, knocking him unconscious and, in a life-or-death situation, breaking the spinal cord. In the latter case, it could be that the assailant has a knife and is intent on thrusting it in the defender's abdomen, thus necessitating a severe response. Note that this defense works equally well from a punching or grabbing attack. It is not confined to being a response to a wrist grab. Herein lies the value of proper bunkai.

Scenario: Attacker grasps you by the opposite wrist and attempts to pull you to another area, into a vehicle or into a punch or strike with the other hand.

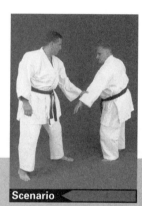

Scenario

Tactics:

1 Step away from the attacker's free hand while at the same time raising your captured wrist high, exposing the back of the attacker's grasping arm.

2 Immediately drive a knifehand strike into the Tw.12 point in the middle of the triceps muscle. The reflexive reaction will cause the attacker to buckle at the knees and bend forward.

Continued on page 120.

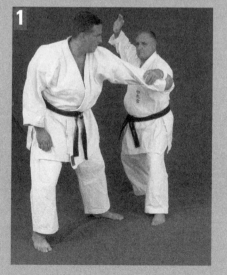

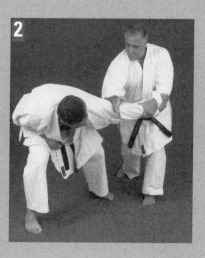

3 Without hesitation, kick hard into the Gb.24/25 or Li.13/14 points on and around the floating ribs. This kick can easily break the ribs and incapacitate the assailant.

4 If the attacker is not dissuaded, jump forward and, using your whole body weight, slam your fore-arm once more into the attacker's

Tw.12 point to knock him to his knees, punch downward to Gb.20 or St.5 at the side of the attacker's jaw, or strike any other offered target to stun or knock him out.

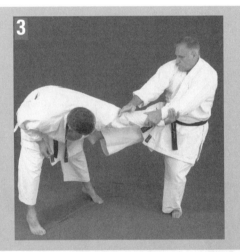

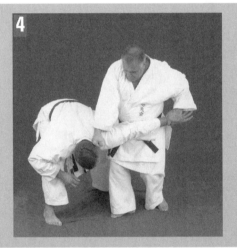

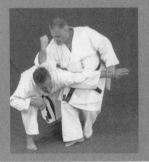

Variation: In a life-threatening situation, the coup de grace is delivered by jumping into the air and driving your elbow down onto the back of the attacker's neck to damage the cervical vertebrae, which can cause paralysis or death.

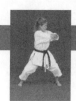

Empi (Elbow Strike), Gedan Barai (Down Block), throw, Otoshi Zuki (Punch)

Scenario: *Assume the guard posture with both hands open, palms towards the attacker. The attacker throws a right punch.*

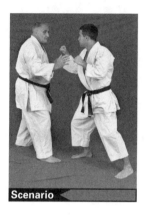

Scenario

Tactics:

1-2 Perform a frisbee *uke*, immediately followed by a roundhouse elbow strike to the attacker's face to stun him. If the attack ceases at this stage, leave the scene.

3 If the attack continues, grasp the back of the attacker's neck with the same hand that delivered the frisbee *uke*, at the same time seizing the attacker's punching arm with the other hand. Pull the attacker's head and body strongly into your own body.

Continued on page 122.

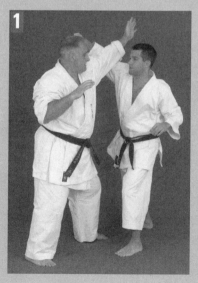

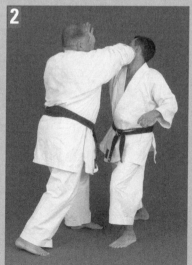

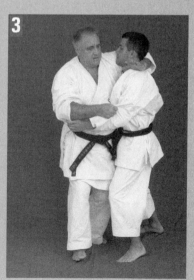

4-5 At the same time, pivot on your right leg, with the left stepping around in a circular movement across the attacker's legs to throw him down to the ground at your feet.

6 While holding firmly with your left hand, deliver a finishing strike with your right.

Using the vital points facilitates this technique in the following way: The first defensive movement (frisbee *uke*) will slam into the vital points on the attacker's arm, causing pain and a slight buckling of the knees, which will allow time for the elbow strike to be delivered to the face. The fluid shock delivered by this blow will cause the brain to be driven against the inside of the skull to stun the assailant. This effect is then magnified by using the same arm that reached around the attacker's neck to be driven firmly into the Gb.20 point on the back of the neck, which will also create a stunning effect. With the opponent on the ground, the final strike anywhere on the face or the side of the head will ricochet the skull into the ground and once again cause the brain to impact against it, causing unconsciousness.

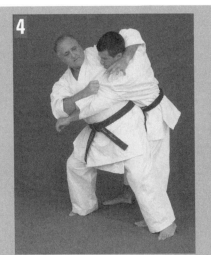
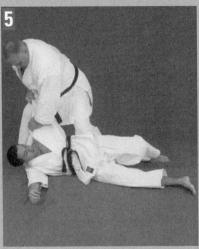
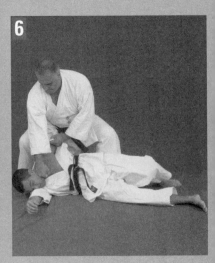

Nijushiho

Originally known as Ni-seishi, the kata is now best known for its use of the side-thrust kick. This, however, is a later introduction and is normally used to demonstrate flexibility rather than defensive prowess. The kata is a significant repository of some excellent defensive *bunkai*.

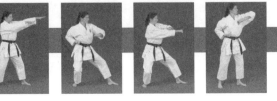

Opening moves: *Kamae (both hands raise defensively), Otoshi Teisho (Dropping Palm Heel), Gyaku Zuki (Punch), Empi Uchi (Elbow Strike)*

Scenario: *The attacker seizes your right wrist with his left hand while preparing to throw a punch to your head with his right.*

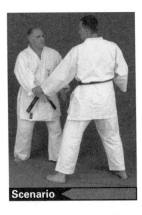

Scenario

Tactics:

1 Immediately extend your left hand and thrust it into the attacker's throat (Cv.22 point) while simultaneously raising the other hand. This combination will invoke a reflexive withdrawal response in the attacker as well as straighten his gripping arm, exposing the next point in the sequence to be struck, Lu.5.

2-3 Pull back your left hand to strike the forearm point (Lu.5). This will force the attacker to release his grip, enabling you to punch the side of the attacker's jaw (St.5 point) or directly to the point of the jaw to deliver a massive shock to the brain. The blow to the Lu.5 point will also cause the attacker to buckle at the knees and bend forward, moving his head directly into the path of the oncoming punch, thus multiplying the impact power. This will stun the attacker and cause him to pull his head backwards.

4 Apply a knockout strike with the elbow of the other arm to the side of the attacker's head or jaw.

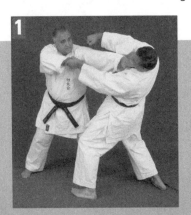

1

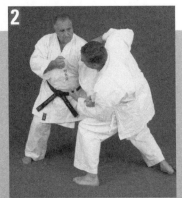

2

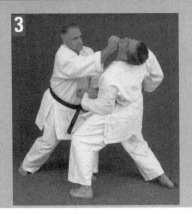

3

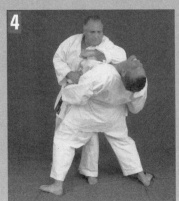

4

Age Uke (Upward Block), Age Empi (Elbow Strike), Tate Shuto Uke (Upright Knifehand Block), Yokogeri Kekomi (Side Kick), Chudan Zuki (Punch)

Scenario: The attacker assumes a boxing-type stance and throws a punch to your head.

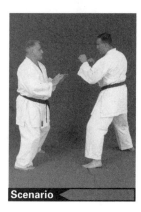

Scenario

Tactics:

1-2 Immediately perform a frisbee *uke* block using the arm on the same side as the attacker's punching arm; continue directly with an upward elbow strike with the other arm to any part of the attacker's chin or face.

3 In a continuing rapid sequence, slide your left blocking arm under the attacker's armpit and pull it towards you, then strike hard (using a hammerfist or knifehand strike) to the Gb.20 point on the back of the attacker's neck with the other fist to stun or knock him unconscious.

Continued on page 126.

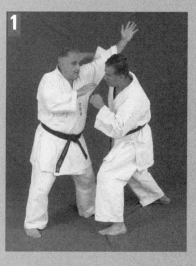

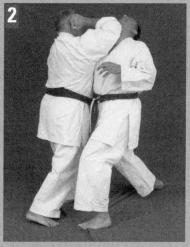

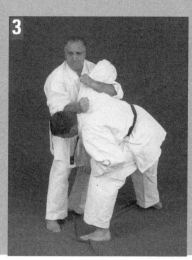

4 From this moment, the attacker should be rendered at the very least extremely dizzy, but if necessary he can be finished off and moved out of the way by driving a kick into the spleen point Sp.11 on the inside of his thigh. This will force his body to buckle and move away from you.

5-7 Deliver a knee strike to the attacker's head and, seizing his head with one hand, twist his body sharply downward. Pull his head down while levering him forward with your left arm and throw him to the ground.

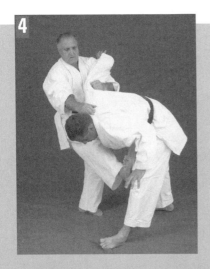

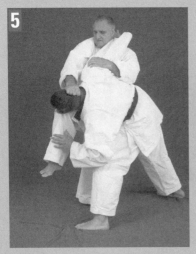

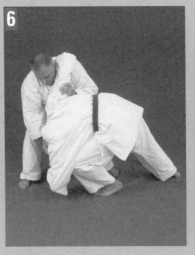

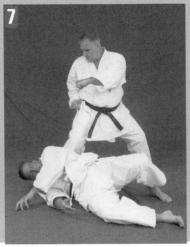

INDEX

Recommended Reading

Any work (books, magazine articles) by Harry Cook

Comprehensive Applications of Shaolin Chin Na: The Practical Defense of Chinese Seizing Arts for All Styles by Yang Jwing-Ming (Yang's Martial Arts Association: Jamaica Plain, MA; 1995)

The History of Karate: Okinawan Goju-Ryu by Morio Higaonna (Dragon Books: Thousand Oaks, CA; 1998)

Karate Jutsu: The Original Teachings of Gichin Funakoshi by Gichin Funakoshi, translated by John Teramoto (Kodansha International: Tokyo; 2001)

Jui Jitsu & Kuatsu by Graham J. Rennie (International Jui Jitsu Academy PTY Ltd.: Brisbane, Australia; 1974**)**

Okinawa Island of Karate by George W. Alexander (Yamazato Publications: Lake Worth, FL; 1991)

Pressure Point Fighting: A Guide to the Secret Heart of Asian Martial Arts by Rick Clark (Tuttle Publishing: North Clarendon, VT; 2001)

The following titles are available at www.kissakikarate.com:
Kyusho Secrets by Vince Morris (PBS: Nottingham, England; 1998)

LETS Defensive Tactics by Vince Morris (Kissaki-Kai: Marlton, NJ; 2007)

Rules of Combat by Vince Morris (PBS: Nottingham, England; 2000)

A list of DVDs covering the *bunkai* of many kata and also defensive tactics is also available.

Special Note: The author is preparing a DVD that will show in detail the techniques in this book plus provide extra information. You'll be able to follow the precise methods of applying the combat applications effectively. Details available are from www.kissakikarate.com or email: info@kissaki-kai.com.

Other Ulysses Press Books

Complete Krav Maga: The Ultimate Guide to Over 200 Self-Defense and Combative Techniques
Darren Levine and John Whitman, $21.95
Dozens of easy-to-learn, effective hand-to-hand combat moves, weapons defense techniques and a complete physical conditioning workout program.

Plyometrics for Athletes at All Levels: A Training Guide for Explosive Speed and Power
Neal Pire, $15.95
Provides an easy-to-understand explanation of why plyometrics works, the research behind it, and how to integrate it into a fitness program.

Workouts from Boxing's Greatest Champs
Gary Todd, $14.95
Features dramatic photos, workout secrets and behind-the-scenes details of Muhammad Ali, Roy Jones, Jr., Fernando Vargas and other legends.

The Martial Artist's Book of Yoga
Lily Chou with Kathe Rothacher, $14.95
A great training supplement for martial artists, this book illustrates how specific yoga poses can directly improve one's martial arts abilities.

Forza: The Samurai Sword Workout
Ilaria Montagnani, $14.95
Transforms sword-fighting techniques into a program that combines the excitement of sword play with a heart-pumping, full-body workout.

Functional Training for Athletes at All Levels: Workouts for Agility, Speed and Power
James C. Radcliffe, $15.95
Teaches athletes the exercises that will produce the best results in their sport by mimicking the actual movements they utilized in that sport.

Total Heart Rate Training: Customize and Maximize Your Workout Using a Heart Rate Monitor
Joe Friel, $14.95
Shows anyone participating in aerobic sports how to increase the effectiveness of his or her workout by utilizing a heart rate monitor.

To order these books call 800-377-2542 or 510-601-8301, fax 510-601-8307, e-mail ulysses@ ulyssespress.com, or write to Ulysses Press, P.O. Box 3440, Berkeley, CA 94703. All retail orders are shipped free of charge. California residents must include sales tax. Allow two to three weeks for delivery.

About the Author and Photographer

Vince Morris is a former judoka and long-time student of Shiro Asano, 9th *dan* and chief instructor of Shotokan Karate International (SKI) in Great Britain and Europe. Vince was a constant member of the Honbu British and European Championship–winning "A" team and the SKI European squad in both *kumite* and kata. On the political front, Vince served as the chairman of the Martial Arts Commission, overseeing all martial arts in England. When the Federation of Shotokan Karate (FSK) was asked to represent England at the 1990 Japanese Karate Association's World Championships in Dubai, Vince was selected as the team coach.

For many years Vince has researched the origins of modern techniques and the applications of kata. His book *The Karate-Do Manual* (1979) introduced the use of the phrase Kyusho Jutsu ("vital point techniques"), shifting the focus away from the relatively new sports-oriented style of karate exemplified by Shotokan and delving into a deeper study of the original concepts and practical effectiveness of traditional karate.

Developing his connections with military and law-enforcement training, he continues to research and refine his teaching, dividing the emphasis equally between the promotion of the health-giving and character-building sporting side of martial arts and that area devoted to cultivating the pragmatic and reliable control and protection techniques for which his training is well known. Vince eventually formed Kissaki-kai Karate-Do in 1993, committed to re-introducing the original principles and values of real karate. With member dojos all over the world, Kissaki-Kai has now established a *honbu* dojo in New Jersey.

Vince continues to produce books (among them, *The Rules of Combat*, *Kyusho Secrets* and *Karate for Kids*), DVDs (including a series of kata *bunkai* videos) and magazine articles promoting the importance of a realistic approach to the martial arts and has just published a law-enforcement training manual. He continues to travel the world presenting seminars. For more details, visit www.kissakikarate.com.

Sensei Billy Bly began studying martial arts in the mid-1970s and became quite serious while working as a bouncer and armed guard. He attended Rochester Institute of Technology, where he studied industrial engineering, criminal justice, and art and design. In 1981 he moved to NYC, where he began studying photography; he also began traveling to photograph nature, especially pelagic birds. A leg injury gave reason to find different work. In 1994 he moved to Europe to join his wife, who was on mission with the United Nations during the war after the split of Yugoslavia. While in Europe, he combined photographic skills and martial arts, traveling the world to cover events. Returning from Europe in 1997, he began *American Samurai*, which started as a dojo and has evolved into a quarterly magazine and monthly newsletter. Sensei Bly is well known for his ability to catch the moment in action photography. His work appears regularly in national publications. He and his son, along with others, have managed to bring traditional martial arts locally through the dojo in Raleigh, NC, where classes are offered in karate and judo. Sensei Bly has black belts in both judo and karate but considers himself a student always. He is eager to learn from his many colleagues and has a simple motivation to try and "make a difference."